medicine

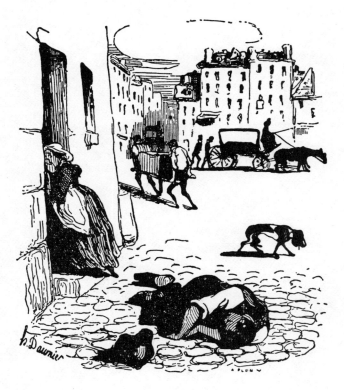

CHARLES E. ROSENBERG

THE CHOLERA YEARS

The United States in 1832, 1849, and 1866

CHICAGO AND LONDON

THE UNIVERSITY OF CHICAGO PRESS

THE UNIVERSITY OF CHICAGO PRESS, CHICAGO 60637
The University of Chicago Press, Ltd., London

89 88 87 86 85   8   9   10   11

ISBN: 0-226-72678-9 (clothbound); 0-226-72679-7 (paperbound)

Library of Congress Catalog Card Number: 62-18121

For Laura

ACKNOWLEDGMENTS

I should like to express my indebtedness to Richard Hofstadter for his guidance in the completion of this book. I am grateful as well to Dumas Malone, David Donald, and Robert Cross for their criticism and encouragement. I was, moreover, fortunate in being able to turn for counsel in matters medical to Owsei Temkin of Johns Hopkins University.

I wish to acknowledge as well the generous financial aid of the Woodrow Wilson Foundation, Columbia University, and the National Institutes of Health. I have also benefited from the encouragement of friends, especially Paul Cranefield, Charles N. Glaab, and Gerald Gruman, whose comments and suggestions have saved me from errors both of style and content.

The publisher of the *Bulletin of the History of Medicine* has kindly given permission for the inclusion of material which originally appeared in that journal.

I owe an especial debt of gratitude to Erwin H. Ackerknecht, of the University of Zürich, who introduced me to the social aspects of medical history and without whose encouragement and inspiration this book would never have been written. My wife Carroll has helped me constantly and thoughtfully.

Madison, Wisconsin

CONTENTS

ix

Part 3

1866

XI   THE METROPOLITAN BOARD OF HEALTH   192

XII   THE GOSPEL OF PUBLIC HEALTH   213

XIII   CONCLUSION: THE WAY WE LIVE NOW   226

       ANNOTATED BIBLIOGRAPHY   235

       INDEX   253

INTRODUCTION

There has not been an active case of cholera in the United States for almost fifty years, and to the present-day American physician it is no more than a chapter in a textbook of tropical medicine. To his nineteenth-century counterpart it was a soul-trying and sometimes fatal reality.

Cholera was the classic epidemic disease of the nineteenth century, as plague had been of the fourteenth. When cholera first appeared in the United States in 1832, yellow fever and smallpox, the great epidemic diseases of the previous two centuries, were no longer truly national problems. Yellow fever had disappeared from the North, and vaccination had deprived smallpox of much of its menace. Cholera, on the other hand, appeared in almost every part of the country in the course of the century. It flourished in the great cities, New York, Cincinnati, Chicago; it crossed the continent with the forty-niners; its victims included Iowa dirt farmers and New York longshoremen, Wisconsin lead miners and Negro field hands.

Before 1817, there had probably never been a cholera epidemic outside the Far East; during the nineteenth century, it spread through almost the entire world.[1] Of all epidemic dis-

[1] Though there is some controversy as to the extent of cholera's early peregrinations, most historians of the disease agree that it has been endemic only

eases, only influenza in the twentieth century has had a more extensive odyssey.

Cholera could not have thrived where filth and want did not already exist; nor could it have traveled so widely without an unprecedented development of trade and transportation. The cholera pandemics were transitory phenomena, destined to occupy the world stage for only a short time—the period during which public health and medical science were catching up with urbanization and the transportation revolution. Indeed, cholera was to play a key role in its own banishment from the Western world; the cholera epidemics of the nineteenth century provided much of the impetus needed to overcome centuries of governmental inertia and indifference in regard to problems of public health.

It was not easy for survivors to forget a cholera epidemic. The symptoms of cholera are spectacular; they could not be ignored or romanticized as were the physical manifestations of malaria and tuberculosis. One could as easily ignore a case of acute arsenical poisoning, the symptoms of which are strikingly similar to those of cholera.[2] The onset of cholera is marked by diarrhea, acute spasmodic vomiting, and painful cramps. Consequent dehydration, often accompanied by cyanosis, gives to the sufferer a characteristic and disquieting appearance: his face blue and pinched, his extremities cold

---

in India, especially in the Ganges River Valley. A recent and inclusive outline of cholera's history may be found in R. Pollitzer, *Cholera* (Geneva, 1959), pp. 11–50. Still important are August Hirsch, *Handbuch der historisch-geographischen Pathologie*, Bd. I, *Die allgemeinen acuten Infectionskrankheiten* (Stuttgart, 1881), pp. 278–348, and Georg Sticker, *Abhandlungen aus der Seuchengeschichte und Seuchenlehre*, Bd. II, *Die Cholera* (Giessen, 1912). The only general account of cholera in the United States is that by J. S. Chambers, *The Conquest of Cholera* (New York, 1938). This is based on the monumental United States government report on cholera prepared between 1873 and 1875 by John Shaw Billings, Ely McClellan, and John C. Peters, *The Cholera Epidemic of 1873 in the United States*, 43d Cong., 2d sess., Doc. 95 (Washington, 1875).

[2] A cholera epidemic provided an ideal occasion for the removal of unwanted spouses, affluent and immoderately aged uncles, and the like. See, for example, *Boston Medical and Surgical Journal*, VII (February 15, 1832), 20; *Herald* (New York), August 14, 1849; *Sun* (New York), August 2, 1849.

and darkened, the skin of his hands and feet drawn and puckered. "One often," recalled a New York physician, "thought of the Laocoön, but looked in vain for the serpent." Death may intervene within a day, sometimes within a few hours of the appearance of the first symptoms. And these first symptoms appear with little or no warning. He felt no premonition of cholera at all, reported a New Yorker in 1832, until he pitched forward in the street, "as if knocked down with an axe."[3]

The abrupt onset and fearful symptoms of cholera made Americans apprehensive and reflective—as they were not by the equally deadly, but more deliberate, ravages of tuberculosis or malaria. "To see individuals well in the morning & buried before night, retiring apparently well & dead in the morning is something which is appalling to the boldest heart."[4] It is not surprising that the growing public health movement found in cholera an effective ally.

It was not until 1883 that Robert Koch, directing a German scientific commission in Egypt, isolated the organism that causes cholera—*Vibrio comma*, a motile, comma-shaped bacterium. Once they find their way into the human intestine, these vibrios are capable of producing an acute disease which, if untreated, kills roughly a half of those unfortunate enough to contract it.[5] Cholera, like typhoid, can be spread along any pathway leading to the human digestive tract. Unwashed hands or uncooked fruits and vegetables, for example, are frequently responsible for the transmission of the disease, though sewage-contaminated water supplies have been the

[3] Edward H. Dixon, *Scenes in the Practice of a New York Surgeon* (New York, 1855), p. 15; John Stearns to the New York City Board of Health, July 19, 1832, Filed Papers of the Common Council, File Drawer T-592, Municipal Archives and Records Center.

[4] Diary of a Young Man in Albany, July 18, 1832, Manuscript Division, New York Historical Society.

[5] In Russia in 1921, for example, there were some 207,000 cases with a mortality of 44.8 per cent (Richard P. Strong, *Stitt's Diagnosis, Prevention, and Treatment of Tropical Diseases* [Philadelphia, 1944], II, 592).

cause of the most severe, widespread, and explosive cholera epidemics.

Though never endemic in this country, cholera returned to the United States four times after its initial appearance in 1832–34. After this two-year visit, North America was free of the disease until the winter of 1848–49. Between 1849 and 1854, however, no twelve-month period passed without cholera appearing in some part of the United States. Then the disease disappeared as abruptly as it had in 1834; it was not to return until 1866.[6]

Thirty-four years are a short time in man's history. Yet few historians would question the significance or magnitude of the changes effected in American society between 1832 and 1866. Comparatively little, however, has been written in a systematic attempt to define the dimensions of this social change or to describe the nature of the processes which brought it about. The following pages attempt not simply to describe three epidemics, but to understand something of America in the cholera years—in 1832, 1849, and 1866.

In point of numbers, few Americans actually died of cholera: for each of its victims, malaria and tuberculosis claimed scores. Unlike them, however, it was novel and terrifying, a crisis demanding response in every area of American life and thought. I have sought to make the cholera epidemics serve as sampling technique as well as subject. They represented a constant and—in the sense that cholera was never endemic in the United States—randomly recurring stimulus against which the varying reactions of Americans could be judged.

Perhaps most striking of the changes in America between 1832 and 1866 was the dissipation of the piety still so characteristic of many Americans in the Age of Jackson. The evangelical fervor of this earlier generation had been eroded by a

---

[6] It appeared again in 1873, but was on this occasion limited almost exclusively to the Mississippi River Valley. It was feared in 1881–83 and 1892 that cholera would again be imported. On neither occasion, however, did it establish itself in this country.

materialism already present in 1832, but seemingly triumphant by 1866. Habits of thought and patterns of rhetoric had changed as well. A more critical and empirical temper had begun to replace the abstract rationalism of an earlier day. In medicine, for example, thoughtful physicians scorned those concepts which could not be expressed in tables and percentages. The most skeptical disavowed traditional therapy and relied upon the body's natural powers to triumph over disease.[7] This "positivistic" temper of thought and expression infiltrated the pulpit and editorial page as well as the laboratory and consultation room. Cholera, a scourge of the sinful to many Americans in 1832, had, by 1866, become the consequence of remediable faults in sanitation. Whereas ministers in 1832 urged morality upon their congregations as a guarantor of health, their forward-looking counterparts in 1866 endorsed sanitary reform as a necessary prerequisite to moral improvement.[8] There could be no public virtue without public health.

[7] Those medical men who dogmatically denied the efficacy of all remedies not validated "numerically," were termed by contemporaries "therapeutic nihilists." Cf. Erna Lesky, "Von den Ursprüngen des therapeutischen Nihilismus," *Sudhoffs Archiv*, XLIV (1960), 1–20; Walter Artelt, "Louis' amerikanische Schüler und die Krise der Therapie," *ibid.*, XLII (1958), 291–301; Erwin H. Ackerknecht, "Die Therapie der Pariser Kliniker zwischen 1795 und 1840," *Gesnerus*, XV (1958), 151–63.

[8] It might be argued that this picture is overdrawn, that if another disease were to be studied, smallpox let us say or syphilis, very different conclusions might be reached. A student of the history of smallpox, for example, might conclude that theistic explanations of disease had almost disappeared by 1832. Yet, as is apparent, this would not be attributable to any necessary decrease in individual piety, but to a somewhat fortuitous advance in scientific knowledge (that is, vaccination) which made such explanations increasingly irrelevant. In the case of venereal disease, on the other hand, very different factors were at work; the emotion-laden response of even physicians to its sexual mode of transmission helped preserve the moralistic attitudes with which such ills were regarded until well into the twentieth century. There is no necessary contradiction in these conclusions; moralism is not piety and smallpox is not syphilis. A disease is no absolute physical entity but a complex intellectual construct, an amalgam of biological state and social definition. The reactions of Americans to cholera changed between 1832 and 1849, between 1849 and 1866. This is unquestionable. My task has been to understand something of the factors which enabled Americans to perceive this old phenomenon in a new way.

The means of improving the public health seemed clear enough. Clean streets, airy apartments, a pure supply of water, were certain safeguards against epidemic disease. And by 1866, advocates of sanitary reform could in justification of their programs point to the discovery of John Snow, a London physician, that cholera was spread through a contaminated water supply.[9] The matter-of-fact, empirical approach to epidemiology which enabled Snow to confirm his theory of the disease's transmission would have been rare a century before. He had, as well, new theories of disease causation, of the very nature of disease, available to him. Cholera in 1849, for example, was assumed by the great majority of physicians to be a specific disease, whereas in 1832, most practitioners had still regarded cholera as a vague atmospheric malaise and had vigorously disavowed the very existence of specific disease entities.

In 1832, most Americans regarded the United States as a land of health, virtue, and rustic simplicity. Cities seemed often unnatural and perhaps ultimately undesirable excrescences in our otherwise green and pleasant realm. By 1866, this was no longer the case. America's cities had grown immensely in size and significance; they could be deplored, but no longer ignored. But though the existence of the city might be inevitable, its evils were not. The willingness to accept the city and its continued growth was an indispensable step in the finding of appropriate solutions to the problems such growth created. Flight to the country was no longer in 1866, as it had been to many in 1849, an acceptable solution to urban problems. A pure water supply, adequate sanitation, and a reliable police force were necessary if the dangerous and unhealthful conditions of city life were to be ameliorated.

[9] Snow originally published his theory of the mode of communication of cholera in 1849. It was not until the London cholera epidemic of 1854, however, that he was able to prove empirically his earlier assertions. Snow's writings on cholera have been conveniently reprinted under the auspices of the Commonwealth Fund, *Snow on Cholera, Being a Reprint of Two Papers by John Snow, M.D. . . .* (New York, 1936).

When in the spring of 1832 Americans awaited cholera, they reassured themselves that this new pestilence attacked only the filthy, the hungry, the ignorant. There seemed few such in the United States. In the spring of 1866, when Americans again prepared themselves for an impending cholera epidemic, they expected no such exemption. North America had nurtured slums as squalid as any of those festering in the Old World. Their inhabitants, moreover, were not the pious, cleanly, and ambitious Americans of an earlier generation. Filthy, illiterate peasants could expect no greater exemption from cholera in Boston than that which they had received in Ireland. America was no longer a city set upon a hill. The piety which sustained such a belief and the confidence which this belief engendered were both disappearing. Americans were adjusting to life on the plain.

These remarks are, I hope, sufficient to suggest the kinds of problems dealt with in the following pages. The body of this study is divided into three sections, corresponding to the three major cholera outbreaks on American soil. Each section is intended to be self-sufficient, and all are roughly parallel in organization. Inclusions and omissions which may seem arbitrary in any one of the three sections have been dictated by the design of the work as a whole.

Social attitudes reflect needs as well as realities, wish as well as fulfilment. Many of the ideas outlined in the following pages are inconsistent, even contradictory; rarely do they correspond accurately to the realities of American life, for men perceive their world through a glass darkened by the particular assumptions and predispositions of their generation. Yet popular convictions must not be dismissed as merely crude, or inconsistent, or even irrational.[10] The ideas which

---

[10] Compare the remarks of Pieter Geyl on the problem of irrationality in the causation of the American Civil War, *Debates with Historians* (New York, 1958), chap. xii, "The American Civil War and the Problem of Inevitability," pp. 244–63.

men have held in the past become, through their belief, truth —at least historical truth.

Not that every American, or even any particular American, in 1832, 1849, or 1866 believed in all those ideas which I suggest as typical of their time. Indeed, many were opposed, implicitly or explicitly, to the predominately Protestant and "middle-class" assumptions of their generation. Yet these values were the accepted, the official ones of nineteenth-century America.

A final apology. Much of the narrative portion of this study, as well as many of the illustrative examples of other sections, is drawn from the experience of New York City during the cholera epidemics. This is due only partially to the relative abundance and accessibility of sources describing New York's bouts with cholera. Rather than spending scores of pages in the repetitious chronicling of cholera in city after city, it seemed more profitable to sketch in greater detail the story of these epidemics in one community. And New York was not just another community; it was the largest and most important city in North America.

The sources for this study are varied, though almost half of the research was done in contemporary newspapers and periodicals. For each of the cholera years, at least one hundred newspapers have been consulted. These were chosen in the hope of arriving at a balanced sampling of opinion, urban and rural, northern and southern, secular and denominational. Periodicals, far less numerous than newspapers in mid-nineteenth-century America, have been examined whenever available.

Perhaps a fourth of the material used in this book was gleaned from medical sources. These include medical journals, treatises, casebooks, and the like. With almost nothing known of cholera and its cause, physicians, especially in 1832 and 1849, clearly reflected the values and preconceptions of their class and time in the discussion of what are ostensibly medical problems. A careful study of their writings on cholera discloses as well something of the slow and complex way in which scientific ideas change, not necessarily in the minds of a few great men, but in that substrate of assumption and accepted wisdom which constitutes the intellectual texture of an age.

PART I

1832

I. THE EPIDEMIC: 1832

It had been an unhealthy winter and the dry spring promised a sickly summer. But New York, a vigorous city of almost a quarter of a million, had other concerns in the spring of 1832. She was the greatest port of the continent, one of the greatest in the world, and her leaders were busy at wharves and in counting rooms ensuring her continued eminence. It was an election year, and the readers of New York's score of newspapers were not allowed to forget the Indian troubles, the tariff controversy, or the bank question.

Like Boston, Philadelphia, and Baltimore, New York was a city which faced Europe, and there was disquieting news from across the Atlantic. Cholera had broken out in England; a *cordon sanitaire*—enforced by heavily armed troops—had failed to halt the spread of the disease westward from Poland and Russia. Quarantine restrictions seemed to be of no avail, and as the summer of 1832 approached, it appeared more than likely that America, like Russia, France, and England, would be visited by this newest judgment. Only the Atlantic Ocean continued to protect the United States.

This, the first invasion of Europe by cholera, had not gone unnoticed in America. Throughout the fall and winter of 1831–32, newspapers, magazines, and pamphlets reported in alarming detail its westward spread. Most dismaying, because most dispassionate, were the reports of the French and English medical commissions sent to study the disease in Russia and Poland. American medical men turned to the treatises of East India Company physicians, familiar for decades with this pestilence new to the medical world of Europe, in hopes of finding some remedy. By July of 1832, it seemed questionable whether a single periodical had appeared in the past six months without "something on this all engrossing subject."

Private citizens were not alone in their concern. On September 6, 1831, the New York City Board of Health had resolved that three of the city's most prominent physicians be requested to form a committee of correspondence to gather information. In January, Martin Van Buren, minister to the Court of St. James, began sending home reports of the epidemic which had just broken out in Sunderland. In February, the Massachusetts Medical Society appointed a committee of seven to study the history of the disease in an attempt to discover how it might best be treated and whether or not it was contagious.[1]

Collecting information could not alone prevent disease. Stringent quarantines were immediately invoked against Europe's cholera-ridden ports. In the past, restrictions had been applied only during the summer months. But cholera, unlike yellow fever, seemed to show no preference for warm climates, and quarantine regulations were maintained in America's Atlantic ports throughout the winter of 1831–32. As early as September 17, 1831, Mayor Walter Bowne of New York announced that he had made arrangements for a special depot for quarantined goods. Boston, Philadelphia, Charleston, and Baltimore soon followed suit, quarantining all goods and passengers from infected ports in Russia and the

[1] New York City Board of Health, Minutes, September 6, 1831, Municipal Archives and Records Center (cited hereinafter as Minutes). Later references to the actions of the Board of Health for which no reference is cited may be presumed to have come from these minutes. Martin Van Buren, London, to Edward Livingston, Washington, January 14, 1832, Martin Van Buren Papers (microfilm, Columbia University Library); Massachusetts Medical Society, *A Report on Spasmodic Cholera* . . . (Boston, 1832), p. 1.

Baltic.[2] The British Isles were added to the interdicted areas as soon as it became known that cholera had made its appearance in England.

With the spring of 1832 and the recrudescence of the epidemic in Europe, only the most sanguine remained confident that America would continue to be spared. It was, in the words of one editor, "not only absurd but morally wrong for any man to assert" that cholera would not appear in the United States. Our exemption "would imply little less than a miracle in our behalf," for American commerce with infected ports continued unabated. Even the common folk began to sense omens. All that year, one Washingtonian recalled: "The Sun Rised and Set Red . . . and two Black Spots could be discovered disstint in the Sun."[3]

But Americans were not without consolation. Cholera did not attack all, nor did it seem to be an arbitrary imposition of God. It was subject to natural laws and acted through second causes, attacking only those who had somehow weakened or "predisposed" themselves. Filth, misery, vice, and poverty conspired to produce its unfortunate victims. Few such could be found in a land enjoying those unique blessings granted the United States. The healthy farmers and sturdy mechanics of the United States could, Americans believed, never provide such hecatombs of victims as cholera had claimed from among the pagans, Moslems, and papists of Europe and the East. America had no class to compare with the miserable slum-dwellers of Paris and London or with the brutalized serfs of

---

2 *Boston Medical and Surgical Journal* (cited hereinafter as *BMSJ*), V (September 20, 1831), 97; V (November 15, 1831), 226. A memorial from the New York Board of Health to Congress (Minutes, January 4, 1832), suggesting the appointment of a commission to study the disease in Europe, found much support in medical circles. The petition was reported on adversely by the Commerce Committee, although in doing so, it affirmed the power of the federal government to institute a national quarantine if such were to prove necessary. U.S. Congress, *Cholera Morbus*, 22d Cong., 1st sess., January 20, 1832, House Report 226.

3 *Religious Examiner* (Washington, Ohio), V (1832), 63–64; *Argus* (Albany), June 1, 1832; Diary of Michael Shiner, p. 49, Manuscript Division, Library of Congress.

Nicholas' Russia. Even New England mill hands were as well fed and clothed as any class in the world, their habits perfectly regular and temperate. "With clean persons and clean consciences," Americans were prepared to meet the disease without trembling.

Americans, as they readily acknowledged, were the best educated, the freest, and the most pious of people. No established clergy battened upon them; here, "where reason is free to combat error," the printed word enjoyed its greatest influence. Americans would never lose heart, they reassured themselves, become panic stricken, and like the Paris mob, loot and murder when assailed by the disease. English by inheritance, North Americans could be expected to behave calmly and with valor. An unwavering faith in Christ was a bulwark even more secure. The history of cholera seemed to demonstrate clearly that those countries with fewest Christians had been scourged most severely. America's chastisement would certainly be light, the pious hopefully predicted, for fully one half of the world's evangelical Christians lived within her boundaries.

It did not seem, moreover, that a nation predominately rural could be severely tried. Only in the densely populated cities of the Old World had cholera raged uncontrolled. Rural communities were assured that their pure atmosphere, uncrowded streets, and isolation guaranteed exemption from the disease. Even America's great eastern cities seemed cleaner and their inhabitants of better character than their counterparts in Europe. Boston, in particular, prided herself on the cleanliness, the virtue, the regularity and morality of her citizens. Where, as a Congregational sermonist put it, "on the wide earth is there another to be compared with it in point of cleanliness, health, comfort, intelligence, morals, and most of those things which minister to human happiness and improvement."[4]

[4] Samuel Barrett, *A Sermon Preached in the Twelfth Congregational Church, Boston, Thursday, August 9, 1832* . . . (Boston, 1832), pp. 7, 11.

Nevertheless, few pious Americans dared deny that their nation, despite the great favors granted it by the Lord, still harbored a great many of the sinful and vicious—more than enough to provoke divine judgment. New York seemed especially vulnerable, the largest and filthiest, the most crowded and vice-disfigured of American cities.

Apprehensive New Yorkers took stock of their city and were not reassured by what they saw and smelled. New York was dirty, and dirt seemed to breed disease—not only cholera, but yellow fever, malaria, and every other sort of pestilence. Boston and Philadelphia seemed immaculate country villages by comparison.

The thousands of swine that roamed its streets were the city's shame, but, nevertheless, its only efficient scavengers. The indifference of the Common Council to the problem of sanitation almost necessitated the lenience, if not affection, with which the pigs were treated. Ordinances to control them were passed from time to time, but never enforced. Respectable folk were continually exasperated by the sight of the beasts, some even threatening to shoot them on sight.

Pigs, goats, and dogs did not provide the only street cleaning apparatus. Citizens were required by law to sweep in front of their houses on certain specified days. Dust and rubbish were to be gathered into a pile in the middle of the gutter from which place they were to be collected by the municipality. An item of Tammany graft or inefficiency, this collection was usually neglected; and appropriately, the decomposing mass of filth which adorned the middle of the streets was called "corporation pie" (New Yorkers, it should be noted, ordinarily referred to their municipal government as the Corporation). In any case, most informed citizens agreed, the streets could never be cleaned properly unless an adequate supply of water was introduced into the city.

Four decades of agitation for a municipal water system had

failed to bring results.[5] Few travelers failed to comment on
the poor quality of New York water. A standing joke maintained that city water was far better than any other, since it
served as a purgative as well as for washing and cooking. Most
people were sensible enough not to drink it, except when
forced by poverty or betrayed through inadvertence. Only
the poor used the city pumps. Those who could afford the expense had their water supplied in hogsheads from the "pure"
springs and wells of the countryside.

Foreigners regarded dyspepsia as America's national malady, and an American dinner could easily be an unnerving
experience. Filthy and adulterated food was prepared with
little care or cleanliness in kitchens swarming with flies and
then bolted as rapidly as possible—perhaps in self-defense.
Although cleanliness was appreciated as an abstract virtue, its
observance in practice left much to be desired. A New England physician remarked that not one in five of his patients
bathed or washed their bodies in water once a year.[6] And this
was the wholesome New England countryside. For the city
poor, maintaining any kind of cleanliness was almost impossible. Most lived in tiny unventilated apartments, often with
whole families—and perhaps a few boarders—occupying the
same room, a condition deplored by physicians and moralists
alike. The most miserable and degraded lived in unfinished
cellars, their walls a mat of slime, sewage, and moisture after
every rain. Houses adjoined stables, abattoirs, and soap factories; their front yards were the meeting place of dogs,
swine, chickens, and horses.

Their city a seemingly foreordained stopping place for
cholera, New Yorkers naturally questioned the powers which
their municipal government would be able to call upon should
there be an epidemic. The experience of the city in a series of

[5] For a discussion of these efforts, see Nelson Blake, *Water for the Cities*
(Syracuse, 1956).

[6] [A Physician], *A Rational View of the Spasmodic Cholera* . . . (Boston,
1832), p. 17.

yellow fever epidemics had provided the administrative framework of a public health organization. The temporary health committees of the 1790's had, by 1832, evolved into a permanent Board of Health with accepted powers and duties, which was, however, almost always quiescent unless an epidemic was actually in progress. (The Board of Health consisted of the aldermen meeting with the recorder and mayor, the mayor acting as president of the board and exercising its powers when it was not in session.) In the ten years after the yellow fever epidemic of 1822, the board met at stated but infrequent intervals, although interest was so slight that the necessary quorum was often unobtainable. The Board of Health was charged with the administration and enforcement of the city's public health regulations, which, in practice, consisted almost entirely of enforcing quarantine. The connection between yellow fever in the West Indies or the South and New York's outbreaks of the disease was too obvious to have been ignored. Thus, almost all of the board's stated meetings took place during the summer, when there was danger from the South. The day-to-day business of keeping a city of a quarter of a million healthy was the responsibility of only three men, the health officer of the port, the resident physician, and the city inspector.

The health officer, appointed by the state and working in conjunction with the Board of Health, was responsible for enforcing the quarantine regulations. The duty of the resident physician, a municipal appointee, was to diagnose and report any communicable diseases which might exist in the city. This was a peculiarly vulnerable position, for premature diagnosis of an epidemic disease would mean severe loss to the city's business.[7] The resident physician in 1819 who had had the

[7] This characterization of the Board of Health is drawn primarily from the Minutes of the board, complete for the period June 5, 1829, to November 23, 1836. The Municipal Archives, at which these minutes are deposited, also contains the complete papers of the board for 1832, including some fifteen hundred reports of cases made by physicians. There are a few articles which shed some light on the activities and evolution of the board. See especially

temerity to diagnose a case of yellow fever was bestowed
with "every abusive epithet which could degrade or disgrace"
and threatened with personal injury. (The board itself was, as
William Dunlap remarked to his friend Dr. John W. Francis,
"more afraid of the merchants than of lying.")[8] The city inspector, another municipal officer, was more strictly an ad-
ministrator, charged with the keeping of vital statistics and
the enforcement of sanitary regulations.

The weaknesses of the board were apparent to even the
most casual observer. Composed of laymen, it was dependent
for advice upon the city's physicians, while as an executive
committee, it was dependent upon the Board of Assistant
Aldermen for financial and legislative support. The board had
only three regular employees, a secretary and two assistants.
It had no office, no dispensary, not even a library. It hiber-
nated each winter. Its membership was undistinguished, and as
events were to show, slow to act on professional advice when
it seemed to endanger the financial well-being of the city.

As spring warmed into summer, the inactivity of the Corporation began to provoke more and more criticism. Nothing,
it seemed, had been done to protect the city. Cholera would
rage uncontrollably should it arrive "at this moment," one
critic warned early in June, "in the midst of the filth and
stench with which our streets are filled."[9] But the authorities
had not been completely supine. Walter Bowne, the mayor,
had hastened to proclaim a blanket quarantine against almost
all of Europe and Asia. On June 4, a new act to regulate the
cleaning of the city's streets was introduced into the Board of

George Rosen, "Public Health Problems in New York City during the Nineteenth Century," *New York State Journal of Medicine*, L (1950), 73–79;
Rosen, "Politics and Public Health in New York City (1833–1842)," *Bulletin
of the History of Medicine*, XXIV (1950), 441–61; Charles F. Bolduan, "Public
Health in New York City," *Bulletin of the New York Academy of Medicine*,
2d ser., XIX (1943), 423–41.

[8] William Dunlap, *Diary of William Dunlap (1766–1839)* (New York,
1930), III, 814.

[9] *Truth Teller* (New York), June 2, 1832.

Assistants. The act, which was signed by the Mayor on Wednesday, June 13, completely reorganized New York's sanitation system.[10]

Two days later, on the fifteenth, the threat became more real and more imminent. The Albany steamboat which docked that Friday afternoon brought word that cholera had broken out in Quebec and Montreal. The Atlantic had been forded—America's last great defense had failed, and it hardly seemed possible that she could be spared.

New York was not a large city. By Saturday morning, June 16, nearly everyone had heard the news from Canada. Philip Hone, the usually imperturbable ex-mayor, did not see how New York could escape. He could not think of a European city as dirty as New York; certainly neither Quebec nor Montreal was dirtier.[11] Miasma arising from the filth rotting in the streets, yards, and cellars was quite capable of producing sickness without the added influence of cholera in the atmosphere.

The members of the Common Council were equally conscious of the sights and smells; self-preservation as well as political expendiency demanded their immediate action. On Saturday morning, the Board of Assistants held a special meeting and voted $25,000 to the Board of Health for "the erection of hospitals and other means to alleviate and prevent the cholera." The board was also urged to send a suitable observer to report on the epidemic in Canada. Skilled observation would provide insight and understanding, perhaps even a cure or preventive for the disease.[12]

[10] *Evening Post* (New York), February 3, 1832, reprints the Mayor's quarantine proclamation issued the previous day. New York City, Board of Assistants, *Report of the Committee on Cleaning Streets*, Doc. 36 (New York, 1832).

[11] Diary of Philip Hone, June 15, 1832, Manuscript Division, New York Historical Society. A portion of Hone's comments may be found in Allan Nevins' edition of the Hone Diary, *The Diary of Philip Hone 1828–1851* (New York, 1927), I, 65–66.

[12] N.Y.C. Common Council, *Proceedings of the Board of Assistants, from May 8, 1832 to May 14, 1833* (New York, 1837), II, 33, 36. Doctors DeKay and Rhinelander were sent by the board to observe the disease in Canada.

The news from Canada was uniformly discouraging. The mortality rate in Quebec and Montreal had not been surpassed in any part of the world, and there was little dissent when Mayor Bowne proclaimed an unprecedentedly severe quarantine. Without the permission of the Board of Health, no ship could approach closer than three hundred yards to the city; no vehicle closer than a mile and a half.[13]

It seemed on Sunday that every minister in the city had chosen cholera as his text. "The consternation in the city is universal," a young artist noted in his journal, "Wall Street and the Exchange are crowded with eager groups waiting for the latest intelligence."[14] The Sabbath was profaned by the *Courier and Enquirer*, which printed a cholera extra of ten thousand copies. The *Standard* also issued an extra, while hopeful apothecaries circulated and posted handbills for opium, camphor, and laudanum—all sovereign remedies and preventives for cholera. The price of camphor doubled immediately.

The medical profession was particularly conscious of the danger and of its responsibility should there be an epidemic. Accordingly, the Medical Society, which represented two-thirds of the city's licensed physicians, formed a special committee of fifteen to study the problem. At their first meeting, this committee formulated a program of public and individual hygiene for the days ahead. It was most important, they urged, that the streets be kept clean throughout the coming summer. To help accomplish this, and to purify the atmosphere, water should be run from the hydrants several times a week. The streets themselves, as well as private sinks, yards, and cesspools should be disinfected with chloride of lime or quicklime. Individuals were urged to be calm, to be temperate in dining and drinking, and to be especially scrupulous in washing. Learned in a generation of yellow fever epidemics

13 *Evening Post* (New York), June 16, 1832.

14 Diary of Thomas Kelah Wharton, June 17, 1832, Manuscript Division, New York Public Library.

and gleaned from accounts of cholera in Europe, these recommendations represented the best medical opinion of the time.[15]

Despite such excellent and reassuring advice, many New Yorkers were already leaving or planning to leave the city. Those who stayed stocked up, if they could afford to, on the cholera specifics which were being hurriedly concocted, bottled, and labeled by apothecaries and free-lance quacks. Even the more irreverent were sobered by the threat of this "pestilence that walketh in darkness." The twenty-ninth of June was generally observed as a day of fasting, prayer, and humiliation by the city's numerous congregations. The neighboring city of Brooklyn had observed a similar fast the previous day.[16]

Still, in the face of increasing public concern, the Corporation appeared strangely negligent. To be sure, it had seemed for a few days that the city would be zealous in banishing its filth. A new system of street-cleaning was instituted, and householders were urged individually to clean and purify their buildings and grounds. By the end of the week, however, it was becoming apparent that this ambitious program had come to a halt as abruptly as it had begun. The dirt and rubbish which householders had gathered now lay in ridges in the streets waiting to be carted away. William Cullen Bryant's *Evening Post* (June 22, 23) suggested that the legislature step in to protect the city, the Corporation having proved itself irremediably incompetent.

Cholera appeared in Montreal on June 6. By June 14, it was in Whitehall, New York; by June 18, at Mechanicsville and Ogdensburg.[17]

At the first news of cholera's arrival in Canada, few Ameri-

---

[15] *Truth Teller* (New York), June 23, 1832.

[16] *Observer (New York)*, June 30, 1832.

[17] A detailed survey of the disease's spread through New York State may be found in Lewis Beck, "Report on Cholera, made to his Excellency Gov. Throop, August, 1832," *Transactions of the Medical Society of the State of New York*, 1832–33, pp. 352 f.

cans could continue to hope that their country might long
escape the fate of its northern neighbor. Most of the immigrants who landed in such great numbers in Canada had no
intention of staying, but quickly made their way to the
United States. Despite the assurance of physicians that cholera was not contagious, it was hard to believe that these dirty,
poverty-stricken wanderers did not bring death as well as
hunger and squalor with them.

Bands of American physicians set out immediately for
Quebec and Montreal to study the disease.[18] Few others, however, were willing to chance an encounter with cholera. Roads
leading from Albany, New York, Philadelphia, and other
eastern cities were crowded with families leaving prematurely
for country homes. Towns and cities in upper New York
State, Vermont, and along the Erie Canal invoked quarantine
regulations, but with little success. Emigrants leaped from
halted canal boats and passed the locks on foot, despite efforts
by contingents of armed militia to stop them.

Enos Throop, the governor of New York, had called a
special session of the legislature to meet at noon Thursday,
the twenty-first of June. A committee appointed that afternoon reported a public health bill on Friday morning. In
what may well have been record time, the bill became law,
passed by both houses and signed by the Governor the same
day. The act called for a quarantine between upper and lower
Canada and New York. More important, it empowered each
city and incorporated village not having a board of health
to establish one. In the next few weeks, meetings all over the
state formed boards of health, usually manned by the overseers of the poor and other local officials. Health officers were
appointed, quarantines instituted, and doctors and hostelry
keepers required to report cases of cholera. Householders
were to clean and purify their properties; persistent nuisances
were to be treated as misdemeanors.

[18] Samuel Jackson, Charles Meigs, and Richard Harlan, *Report of the Commission Appointed by the Sanitary Board of the City Councils, To Visit
Canada* . . . (Philadelphia, 1832), p. 37.

New York State was not alone in such hectic preparations, though her needs were most immediate. In every part of the country, communities hastened to form boards of health and to publish recommendations against cholera. Quarantines were established in booming river and canal towns, and indignant letters filled local newspapers, urging the immediate cleansing and purification of streets and alleys. Owners and overseers white-washed slave cabins and stocked medicine chests with cayenne pepper, laudanum, and calomel, which had been recommended as unfailing preventives. Others appealed to God. The faithful gathered in scores of churches, praying and fasting that the Lord might temper his judgment.

New Yorkers anxiously noted the filth accumulating in their streets, the decaying garbage and stagnant pools in vacant lots, and grew even more alarmed as cholera moved steadily south from Montreal and Quebec.[19] Their fears and conjectures were soon to become reality.

Late Monday night, June 26, an Irish immigrant named Fitzgerald came home violently ill. The pain in his stomach grew worse during the night, and in the morning he called a doctor. When the doctor arrived, Fitzgerald was already feeling better, but his two children were sick, complaining of ag-

[19] It is more than likely that cholera was imported into New York independently of the outbreak in Canada. Years later, Dr. Westervelt, the port physician in 1832, stated that "in 1832 cholera arrived in infected ships prior to its outbreak upon the St. Lawrence, but that for prudential motives, the facts were suppressed by the Board of Health. The sick were cared for in the quarantine hospital, and the well emigrants were shipped rapidly from the city." When Ely McLellan was writing his history of cholera in 1874, he attempted to verify Westervelt's story, but found the quarantine records for April, May, and June of 1832 to be missing, while records of preceding and succeeding months were all perfect. *The Cholera Epidemic of 1873 in the United States*, 43d Cong., 2d sess., Doc. 95 (Washington, 1875), pp. 567–68. This is confirmed by Alexander Vache, *Letters on Yellow Fever, Cholera, and Quarantine* . . . (New York, 1852), p. 47 n. In any case, the ship *Brenda* had arrived in Baltimore on the sixth of June after having had fourteen cholera deaths on her passage from Liverpool. *Freeman's Banner* (Baltimore), June 16, 1832; Horatio G. Jameson, "Observations on Epidemic Cholera as It Appeared at Baltimore, in the Summer of 1832," *Maryland Medical Recorder*, III (1832), 372.

onizing cramps in their stomachs. The children died on Wednesday, but not before they were seen by many physicians, all of whom agreed upon a diagnosis of Asiatic cholera.[20] Mrs. Fitzgerald died on Friday, and the next few days brought a scattering of similar cases: patients suffering with intestinal spasms, diarrhea, and vomiting. Most of them died.

By the end of the week, the Board of Health had received several reports of cholera cases. On Friday (June 30), Dr. James Manley, the resident physician responsible for the diagnosis of contagious disease, reported two "undoubted cases."[21] Despite such convincing evidence, the Board of Health and the mayor were still reluctant to make these reports public.

Regardless of official silence, the fact that cholera existed in the city could hardly be kept secret. On his Sunday walk, Philip Hone met the editor of the *Standard*, who had just seen an unmistakable case at the bridewell.[22] Rumors that cholera was moving west and not south from Canada could not stem the growing panic; mass exodus from the city had already begun. A hyperbolic and sarcastic observer remarked later that Sunday had seen "fifty thousand stout hearted" New Yorkers scampering "away in steamboats, stages, carts, and wheelbarrows." Methodists began the prayer meetings which they were to hold every morning that summer from half-past five to half-past six.

[20] N.Y.C. Board of Health, *Reports of Hospital Physicians and Other Documents in Relation to the Epidemic Cholera of 1832*, edited by Dudley Atkins (New York, 1832), pp. 9–10. Statements of witnesses living in 1866, however, affirmed that the first case of cholera occurred on the twenty-first of June in the person of an immigrant who had just arrived from Montreal. *Evening Post* (New York), May 5, 1866.

[21] The original reports may be found in the City Clerk's Papers, File Drawer U-58, Municipal Archives and Records Center. John Stearns, one of the city's most prominent physicians, went to the mayor and begged him to announce that the epidemic had broken out. The mayor, however, denied that the cases reported were anything out of the ordinary. John Stearns, Concerning the Cholera Epidemic, MS 170, Rare Book Room, New York Academy of Medicine.

[22] Diary of Philip Hone, July 1, 1832, Manuscript Division, New York Historical Society.

The Medical Society and its special committee on cholera felt that they could no longer wait upon the dilatory Board of Health—only prompt and decisive action could save the city. On Monday morning (July 2), the Medical Society stated publicly that nine cases of cholera had occurred. Only one had survived.

This announcement was immediately attacked by those New Yorkers who feared—and hoped—that it might have been premature or unwarranted. Unwilling to face the consequences of an epidemic, they turned instinctively against the physicians who had made it impossible to ignore any longer the presence of cholera in the city. The Medical Society was castigated as a private organization usurping the functions of the Board of Health, as a group of private citizens having no authority to make statements affecting the welfare of the entire city. There were many who agreed with banker John Pintard that this "officious report" was an "impertinent interference" with the Board of Health. Had the eager physicians, he asked, any idea of the disaster which such an announcement would bring to the city's business?[23]

Meeting on the same Monday morning, the Board of Health began to take belated measures against the epidemic already in their midst. From that day forward, the board resolved to meet each day at noon. More important, they decided to appoint a select advisory council of seven prominent physicians. This Special Medical Council, a group for which there was neither precedent nor legal sanction, was to become the "brain trust" of the Board of Health, making most of the decisions in fighting the epidemic.

Meanwhile, the equivocal statements of the Board of Health had been more inscrutable than reassuring. The exodus from the city continued. Carts which a few days before had carried merchandise through the streets were now seen loaded

[23] John Pintard, *Letters from John Pintard to His Daughter Liza Noel Pintard Davidson 1816–1833* (New York, 1941), IV, 66.

with the beds, chairs, linen, and tables of families making for
the pure air of the country.

The roads, in all directions, were lined with well-filled stage
coaches, livery coaches, private vehicles and equestrians, all panic
struck, fleeing from the city, as we may suppose the inhabitants
of Pompeii or Reggio fled from those devoted places, when the
red lava showered down upon their houses, or when the walls were
shaken asunder by an earthquake.[24]

By the end of the first week in July, almost everyone who
could afford to had left the city. Farm houses and country
homes within a thirty-mile radius were completely filled.
Roads leading from the city were crowded not only with
carts, horses, and carriages, but with "oceans" of pedestrians,
trudging in the mid-summer heat with packs on their backs.
A merchant living on one of the principal residential streets
recalled that his and one other family were the only ones on
the street to remain. The young wife of another merchant
baked all the bread and cake eaten in her house during the
epidemic—at the end of the summer even making the yeast.
Visitors to the city were struck by the deathly silence of the
streets, unaccustomedly clean and strewn with lime. Even on
Broadway, passers-by were so few that a man on horseback
drew curious faces to upper windows. One young woman
recalled seeing tufts of grass growing in the little-used thor-
oughfares.

   The Fourth of July proved to be an unnaturally quiet one.
Churches were open for divine service, although many pews
were empty, their occupants having left the city. Some ministers had departed as well, heeding the example of their
scattered flocks. Most uncommonly, the "utmost harmony
prevailed during the day, not a single incident occurred."
Cholera had forestalled even the knifings, brawls, and shoot-
ings which customarily adorned the Fourth. The church bells
were silent, and the only noise was that of a "pretty smart can-
nonade of crackers" provided by the boys of the city.

24 *Evening Post* (New York), July 3, 1832.

Nevertheless, the epidemic increased. On Thursday, July 5, the Court of Sessions discharged on their own recognizance all prisoners confined in the almshouse for misdemeanors. Cholera had broken out at the almshouse, and it seemed unjust to expose petty offenders to probable death. The felons in the penitentiary and the bridewell were soon sent to temporary shelters on Blackwells Island.

On Friday the board began to issue daily cholera reports. The appearance of these bulletins at noon soon became the central event of the day, around which besieged New Yorkers built their daily routine. Mornings were given over to speculation about the new report, while afternoons were devoted to discussions of the identity and circumstances of the latest victims. Even the city's score of thriving newspapers were unable to satisfy a seemingly insatiable public curiosity. On Thursday, July 5, the *Gazette* published two extras, one in the morning and one in the afternoon; still, the "run for them was so great that it was impossible to supply the demand."[25]

At last the Board of Health began to take action, outfitting five special cholera hospitals, one in the Hall of Records, another in a school, a third in an old bank, and a fourth in an abandoned workshed. These tardy measures could not still a growing criticism. Had the lives of the city's humble artisans and mechanics been sacrificed to the commercial interests which seemed to have paralyzed the board into inactivity? Editorials urged that the Board of Health be forced to resign if it could not fulfil its duties.[26] The Board itself was becoming desperate: one member—Alderman Meigs—proposed a reward of twenty dollars for any licensed physician who cured a case of cholera (July 14).

Fortunately, the disorganization of the city was never to become complete. Respectable persons of regular habits re-

[25] *Gazette and General Advertiser* (New York), July 6, 1832.

[26] *Cholera Bulletin,* July 9, 13, 1832. This publication was issued twice weekly during the epidemic by "an association of physicians."

assured themselves that they had little to fear. Only the dirty, the intemperate, those who had somehow predisposed themselves, were cholera's intended victims. The Special Medical Council announced on July 10, a day on which there had been forty-five deaths, "that the disease in the city is confined to the imprudent, the intemperate, and to those who injure themselves by taking improper medicines."[27]

Obviously then, the most important task in preventing the spread of cholera was to safeguard the common people against their dangerous habits of life. Accordingly, the Special Medical Council drew up the following recommendations, which were distributed in handbills and published prominently in all of the city's newspapers.

Notice

Be temperate in eating and drinking,

avoid crude *vegetables* and *fruits;*

abstain from *cold water*, when heated;

and above all from *ardent spirits* and

if habit have rendered it indispensable, take much less than usual.

Sleep and clothe warm

Avoid labor in the heat of day.

Do not sleep or sit in a draught of air when heated.

Avoid getting wet

Take no medicines without advice.

As business in the city stagnated, even the most deserving among the poor were soon penniless. In the month of July, the Savings Bank paid out almost $100,000; on one day, Saturday the seventh, over $20,000.[28] On Tuesday, July 16, a

[27] Minutes, July 10, 1832. This communication was ordered printed in all of the city's newspapers. So common were reports of this kind that it is almost impossible to find a newspaper published in one of America's cholera-infected communities which did not, at some time during the summer, contain a similar declaration.

[28] John Pintard, *op. cit.*, IV, 68–69, 73, 75–76.

large meeting at the Merchant's Exchange collected almost
$1,700 for the relief of the poor. Three nights later, another
meeting was held at which $3,811.75 was subscribed, seven-
teen of the city's more prominent merchants giving one hundred dollars apiece. Those who could not give cash were
urged to contribute food or clothing. Distribution and collection centers were established in each of the city's fifteen
wards. By the end of July, this informal Committee of the
Benevolent was providing some five hundred families with
food in one ward alone.

There was never a more delightful exhibition of Christian benevolence than is now witnessed in this city. . . . Numbers of our
most accomplished ladies are engaged day after day in making
garments for the poor and distressed, while Committees of gentlemen . . . are searching out the abode of poverty, filth, and disease, and administering personally to the wants of the wretched
inmates. . . . They have . . . caused the tenements to be white-
washed and cleansed, and the sick to be provided with physicians
or sent to the Hospitals, not omitting to warn the wicked of their
evil ways, and point them to the Great Physician of the Soul.[29]

The Executive Committee of the Board of Health solicited
clothing and food from merchants for use in the hospitals, and
jobs were provided for at least some of those turned out of
work by the epidemic.[30] The city employed additional men
in construction of the new Seventh Avenue. Church groups
set women to work sewing; one church, the Dutch Reformed
at Nassau and Ann streets, supplied work for eighty women
each day.

When Lorenzo Da Ponte arranged for the visit of an Italian
opera company to New York, he could hardly have visualized

[29] Benjamin Cutler, *A Sermon in Behalf of the New-York Protestant Episcopal City-Mission Society* . . . (New York, 1832), p. 16.

[30] N.Y.C. Board of Health, Executive Committee Cashbook, Municipal Archives and Records Center, lists chronologically all the donations which the
board received and their disposition.

their arrival in the midst of a cholera epidemic. Nor could the company have imagined that their first weeks in the New World would be spent lounging on the grass outside a lonely quarantine station. There were few signs of a prospective opera audience on July 30, when Signor Montresor and his troupe of fifty arrived in New York.

There had been thirty-nine deaths that day, and it was common knowledge that many doctors did not even bother to report their cases. Earlier in the week, over a hundred deaths a day had been recorded. Cartloads of coffins rumbled through the streets, and when filled, returned through the streets to the cemeteries. Dead bodies lay unburied in the gutters, and coffin-makers had to work on the Sabbath to supply the demand. Charles G. Finney, the evangelist, recalled having seen five hearses drawn up at the same time at different houses within sight of his door. Harsh smoke from burning clothes and bedding filled the air, mingling with the acrid fumes of burning tar, pitch, and other time-tested preventives. Houses stood empty, prey to dust, burglary, and vandalism. By August, many of the churches were closed—especially those with wealthier congregations. St. George's shut its doors for almost the entire month; its pastor wrote that three-quarters of his flock were absent anyway.

The deserted houses and shops were a constant temptation to the criminal and near-criminal elements of the city, and the Board of Health soon authorized the mayor to employ additional watchmen. Even this did not seem to have been too effective in checking what one newspaperman spoke of as an "epidemic of burglaries." Here, too, was an area for criticism of the municipal authorities.

The cases of housebreaking are numerous, and the plunderers of private dwellings in the wantonness of mischief destroy what they cannot carry away. Carpets are cut to pieces and furniture broken to pieces by these wretches. We hear of persons procuring an insurance against theft, at 5%. The laws, the city regulations, the municipal police ought to be the insurers of the property of every citizen. . . .[31]

Breaking and entering was not the only means of taking advantage of the city's disorganization. Swindlers attempted to defraud the Savings Bank by presenting falsified passbooks, while businessmen were accused of using the epidemic as an excuse for defaulting on their obligations.

The poor, deserving and undeserving, resented the unwonted intrusion of authority into their affairs. As had been the case in epidemics since the Middle Ages, the lower classes forcibly discouraged attempts to take their sick to hospitals, which were regarded as little more than charnel houses. Physicians and city officials were attacked and brutally beaten. Mobs opposed the precipitate burial of the dead that had been dictated by the Special Medical Council. The inmates of one tenement, "a miscellaneous mob of men and women," blocked the hallways of their building, forcing the authorities to lower a coffin out of a window. When it reached the ground, the women of the building stood upon it to prevent its being taken away. They had planned to wake the corpse, and a sizable number of black eyes and bloody noses on both sides testified to the fervor of their convictions.[32]

The Five Points, the city's red-light district, had always been an object of distaste for the respectable, but at no time was their indignation greater than during the epidemic. The case rate was highest in this moral slough, and the disease soon spread to respectable citizens unfortunate enough to live in the vicinity.

The Five Points . . . are inhabited by a race of beings of all colours, ages, sexes, and nations, though generally of but one condition, and that . . . almost of the vilest brute. With such a crew,

[31] *Evening Post* (New York), July 23, 1832. At least some of this vandalism must have stemmed from resentment toward those whose wealth had allowed them to escape the epidemic.

[32] *Commercial Advertiser* (New York), July 3, August 14, 1832.

inhabiting the most populous and central portion of the city, when may we be considered secure from pestilence. Be the air pure from Heaven, their breath would contaminate it, and infect it with disease.[33]

William A. Caruthers, a young Virginia physician and novelist-to-be, helping to treat the poor in the Five Points was shocked at the misery he saw—far worse, he later wrote, than that to be found among the most ill-used of slaves in his native South. The inhabitants of the Five Points seemed to the young physician no longer human. Dead at heart, they endured cholera like "a flock of sheep swept off suddenly by some distemper." Rum was their only anodyne. Loaves of bread distributed by the benevolent had to be cut into quarters, for intact loaves were pawned for drink.[34]

By July 20, the cholera epidemic had reached its height. August brought with it a gradual but steady decline in the number of new cases, and though the epidemic smouldered on throughout that fall, it had completely disappeared by Christmas.

The factors causing its subsidence can, in retrospect, only be guessed at, even by the trained epidemiologist. Almost certainly, however, an important reason was the disappearance of dense concentrations of susceptible persons living in crowded and filthy conditions. Those of the poor who had not died either had some sort of immunity or had been removed by the authorities to less exposed quarters. Changes in the temperature and humidity may have affected either the cholera vibrio or the ability of the water supply to act as a carrier. In any case, cholera's stay in New York was short and left behind no endemic foci from which new epidemics might originate.

[33] *Evening Post* (New York), July 23, 1832. The area was known as the Five Points because it centered on a square at which five streets intersected.

[34] Caruthers, *The Kentuckian in New-York* ... (New York, 1834), II, 28–29.

In the first weeks of August, merchants began to insert notices in the newspapers, announcing that they were open for business and urging the immediate return of those who had fled. The city, they reassured, held no perils for the temperate and prudent. (Still, the Special Medical Council could not declare itself in favor of such a course. It warned those safely ensconced in the country not to risk the fatigue and anxiety of the trip back to the city.) It soon became apparent that the epidemic had spent itself; in the second half of August, the refugees began to trickle back into the city. On August 28, the Special Medical Council pronounced New York safe, and two days later issued its last cholera report. As early as August 20, the Board of Health had begun to close the cholera hospitals, displaying an alacrity conspicuously absent in its preparations for the epidemic. On August 27, the board began to make provisions for the storage and inventory of its remaining supplies. By the end of the month, only one hospital remained open.

With the last days of August, the city began to come fully alive. Some of the "most abominable cowards," it was observed, were already "becoming satirical." John Pintard, who stayed through the whole terrible summer, was pleased at the return of New York to its accustomed animation. His usually acrid prose became almost joyous as he described the resurrected metropolis.

The stores are all open, footwalks lined with bales and Boxes & streets crowded with carts & porters cars. What a contrast to the middle of July when this Bazar of our dry-goods [Pearl Street] had appeared as still & gloomy as the Valley of the Shadow of death, here and there a solitary person standing at the door or leaning across the empty counters mourning over his departed custom. Now all life & bustle, smiling faces, clerks busy in making out Bills, porters in unpacking & repacking Boxes, joy & animation in every countenance.[35]

[35] Pintard, *op. cit.*, IV, 90. This letter is dated August 18, 1832.

But the epidemic had not become a memory for all New Yorkers. William Dunlap wrote on September 3 that more people were dying than when the Corporation reported.[36] And the winter promised to be a severe one: there were hundreds of widows and orphans to be provided for, and beggars could be found in every busy street.

Americans prided themselves on their railroads, canals, and steamboats. Before the end of 1832, cholera was to travel on them all. Few communities, however remote, escaped its visits; and hastily dug graves in every state between Maine and Wisconsin bore witness to the extent of cholera's wanderings. It followed the army of General Scott against Blackhawk, killing white and Indian alike and spreading to Wisconsin and Illinois. So terrifying was the disease that settlers deserted the shelter of Chicago, where it had broken out, preferring to take their chances with the scalping knives of the savages.[37] New York was probably the most thoroughly scourged among the states. Each of the thriving towns along the Erie Canal suffered in its turn, despite quarantines and last-minute attempts at "purification." But it was the immense mortality of the epidemic in New York City that attracted most attention. Accounts soon filled the columns of newspapers in every part of the country; and local governments in New England, the South, and the West absorbed in their turn the abuse and indignation of fellow citizens. What town could boast of its freedom from the filth and decay which invited cholera? Even rural areas contained piles of festering manure and other nuisances capable of attracting the disease.

[36] Dunlap, *op. cit.*, IV, 617.

[37] Harvey E. Brown, *The Medical Department of the United States Army from 1776 to 1873* (Washington, 1873), pp. 149–52; Frank E. Stevens, *The Blackhawk War* (Chicago, 1903), pp. 242–50; and Augustus Walker, "Early Days on the Lakes, with an Account of the Cholera Visitations of 1832," *Publications of the Buffalo Historical Society*, V (1902), pp. 310–15, all contain accounts of General Scott's "cholera campaign."

The larger cities established cholera hospitals, instituted feverish clean-ups, and continued their quarantines. Despite these efforts, only Boston and Charleston among America's larger cities were to escape; New Orleans was probably the most severely visited. Cholera claimed five thousand lives in the Crescent City.[38]

The South was spared until August and September. Some sections, escaping lightly even then, were to be visited with greater severity in the spring of 1833, when the disease, quiescent during the cold of winter, broke out with undiminished virulence in the West and South. Small villages, even isolated farms, were stricken. And here the disease was most terrifying: it had to be faced alone, often without friend, minister, or physician. The appearance of cholera in even the smallest hamlet was the signal for a general exodus of the inhabitants, who, in their headlong flight, spread the disease throughout the surrounding countryside.

Unswayed by the arguments of physicians, common folk insisted that the disease must be contagious. In Chester, Pennsylvania, several persons suspected of carrying the pestilence were reportedly murdered, along with the man who had sheltered them. Armed Rhode Islanders turned back New Yorkers fleeing across Long Island Sound. At Ypsilanti, the local militia fired upon the mail stage from cholera-infested Detroit. Everywhere there were stringent quarantines. The newly arrived foreign immigrants were particularly feared. Even if they did not carry the disease, the dirty and crowded conditions in which they lived and moved provided the perfect soil in which to germinate the seeds of pestilence.

Those who could deserted cities for the pure air and waters of the countryside. Those who could not experimented with

---

[38] Theodore Clapp's *Autobiographical Sketches and Recollections* ... (Boston, 1858), pp. 117–52, contains an excellent account of the epidemic in New Orleans. Cf. Leland A. Langridge, "Asiatic Cholera in Louisiana, 1832–1873" (unpublished Master's thesis, Louisiana State University, 1955). A yellow fever epidemic which raged simultaneously claimed almost as many lives as cholera in the unfortunate city.

other means of prevention. Many dosed themselves with the "cholera preventives" which enriched apothecaries and quacks throughout the country. A greater number took refuge in alcohol; French brandy and port were held in particularly high esteem for their bracing qualities. The more temperate enveloped themselves in camphor vapors, hoping to neutralize the cholera influence which tainted the atmosphere, while many communities hoped to achieve the same end with the fumes of burning tar or pitch. In New Orleans, such clouds of smoke covered whole blocks. No chances could be taken, no possibility ignored. On one Louisiana plantation, the main house was fumigated morning and evening with burning sugar and vinegar, while its inhabitants were enveloped at all times in clouds of dense smoke from tar burning in the yard. Meats were served smothered in garlic, and no one ventured abroad without camphor somewhere on his person.[39]

The epidemic provoked anxiety even in those places fortunate enough to have escaped its effects. Cholera created a peculiar tension—in the words of a young Bostonian, "a state about midway between hope and fear." For some, this tension, added to a life of tedium and hard work, was almost too much to bear. One rural mother, unsure if her son were alive or dead, scrawled in her diary: "Our anxiety increases. The troubles of my life are neither few nor small I have felt today, as tho the brittle thread would not last long."[40] Mothers feared for their young children, even those seemingly healthy. In cholera times, the slightest malaise might be a premonitory symptom of the disease. The country, especially clean and elevated places, seemed to offer the only security against the disease.

Despite many pious hopes, cholera was no converting ordi-

[39] Mary Holley, St. Charles Parish, to her daughter Harrietta, November 10, 1832, Mary Holley Papers, University of Texas, cited in William D. Postell, *Health of Slaves on Southern Plantations* (Baton Rouge, 1951), pp. 76, 78.

[40] Diary of Lucretia Mott Hall, August 12, 1832, Manuscript Division, New York Historical Society.

nance. The vicious seemed merely to have been hardened in their depravity, though the spiritually minded Christian was confirmed in his faith. Deserted streets and desolate towns returned to life with almost indecent haste. Even before the epidemic had run its course, the infidel theaters had opened their doors. In September, Philadelphians applauded Mr. Hackett as a dashing Colonel Nimrod Wildfire, while in New York, Mr. Rice was enjoying his usual success as Jim Crow.

Cholera returned again in 1833 and 1834, then vanished as abruptly as it had come. It was to be fifteen years before it was again to find root in American soil.

II. GOD'S JUSTICE?

Even so disquieting a disease as cholera could not alter existing patterns of thought. It reinforced convictions; it could not change them. To those critical of American society, cholera was the consequence of an unjust social system. To the physician, it was a new and inscrutable threat to be understood and subdued. But to many ordinary householders, it was a consequence of sin; man had infringed upon the laws of God, and cholera was an inevitable and inescapable judgment.

Medical opinion was unanimous in agreeing that the intemperate, the imprudent, the filthy were particularly vulnerable. Cholera was an influence in the atmosphere—debilitating, but malignant only to those who had somehow weakened themselves. And it was not difficult to expose oneself to cholera; the "predisposing" or "exciting causes" were as varied as the occasions for sin. Any imprudence or excess could provoke an attack. In this doctrine of predisposing causes, the needs and attitudes of an awakening science found practical reconciliation with the ancient, and reassuring, idea of sin as a cause of disease. Cholera was a scourge not of mankind but of the sinner.

Faith and reason, religion and science had been interwoven so as to provide a usable context in which to place the epidemic. There was no necessary inconsistency between the doctrine of predisposing causes and that of retribution by the

Lord. At least there did not seem to be. Theology was under-written by the prestige of science, while the injunctions of medicine seemed in perfect accord with the teachings of morality.

Even before cholera had reached this continent, knowledge-able Americans were convinced that only those of irregular habits had anything to fear from the disease. Of "fourteen hundred lewd women" in one street in Paris, newspapers re-ported, thirteen hundred had died of cholera. In some Euro-pean cities, it had been the exception for drunkards to survive a cholera epidemic. It was clear, proclaimed the governor of New York, that "an infinitely wise and just God has seen fit to employ pestilence as one means of scourging the human race for their sins, and it seems to be an appropriate one for the sins of uncleanliness and intemperance. . . ." The editor of one newspaper could not credit letters from Montreal which stated that cholera was beginning to attack the respectable. Not knowing the writer, he could scarcely believe so unlikely a statement.[1]

Once the disease had arrived, it would be too late for the toper or gourmand to reform. A few days of moderation could scarcely undo the physical ravages of a lifetime given over to drink and gluttony. Sexual excess as well left its devotees weakened and "artificially stimulated," their systems defense-less against cholera.[2]

Having finally reached the United States, cholera affirmed such convictions again and again. Dozens of instances seemed to prove that the disease was a scourge almost exclusively of the thoughtless and immoral. Alexander H. Stevens, president of New York's Special Medical Council, reassured fellow citizens by reporting that "the disease had been confined to

[1] New York State, *Messages from the Governors, Comprising Executive Communications to the Legislature* . . . (Albany, 1909), III, 395; *American for the Country* (New York), June 26, 1832.

[2] *Republican* (Nashville), October 29, 1832; *Boston Recorder*, June 27, 1832; Dr. John L. Cobb, *Virginian* (Lynchburg), August 27, 1832.

the intemperate and the dissolute with but few exceptions."
In one house on Laurens Street, thirteen prostitutes had been
attacked, and all but three had died almost immediately. "Not-
withstanding the increase of sickness and death," one observer
noted,

every day's experience gives us increased assurance of the safety
of the temperate and prudent, who are in circumstances of comfort. . . . The disease is now, more than before rioting in the
haunts of infamy and pollution. A prostitute at 62 Mott Street,
who was decking herself before the glass at 1 o'clock yesterday,
was carried away in a hearse at half past three o'clock. The
broken down constitutions of these miserable creatures, perish
almost instantly on the attack. . . . But the business part of our
population, in general, appear to be in perfect health and security.[3]

Whenever any person of substance died of cholera, it was an
immediate cause of consternation, a consternation invariably
allayed by reports that this ordinarily praiseworthy man either
had some secret vice or else had indulged in some unwonted
excess. To die of cholera was to die in suspicious circumstances.[4]

John Pintard, merchant, banker, and founder of the New
York Historical Society, remarked on July 13 that the alarm
in New York City would be great indeed if the disease were
ever to attack the "regular householders." He thanked God
that it remained "almost exclusively confined to the lower
classes of intemperate dissolute & filthy people huddled together like swine in their polluted habitations." A week later,
at the very height of the epidemic, Pintard was still calm.

3 *Mercury* (New York), July 18, 1832.

4 In general, indiscretions in drink and diet were regarded as the most
important predisposing causes: a pineapple or watermelon was a death war-
rant, a dozen oysters, suicide. Overindulgence in alcohol was the most dangerous of all "exciting causes." Though temperance might not save the lives
of confirmed drunkards, yet it would "save their friends the unspeakable
mortification of having it doubted whether Cholera or dissipation was the
cause of their death." *Mercury* (New York), July 18, 1832.

Those attacked were "chiefly of the very scum of the city"; and the sooner this group was dispatched, the sooner the disease would run its course. A newspaper moralist likened cholera to syphilis—scourges created to bring retribution to the transgressor of moral law. Even if New York had to mourn the loss of some estimable citizens, it would be "mere affectation" not to acknowledge that hundreds had been removed "who were festering wounds in the face of society."[5]

Most Americans did not doubt that cholera was a divine imposition. It was a punishment, moreover, coming from God's own hand. "Atheists may deny, but the intelligence and piety, the real wisdom among us, will acknowledge the providence of God; and this acknowledgment will be made by the great majority of our population. They *feel* that God is chastising us."[6] Cholera was a reminder of man's mortality and of God's omnipotence. Pestilence, like war and famine, was, according to most clergymen, a "rod in the hand of God," a final resort of the deity, an appeal to man's fears when there seemed no recourse in appealing to his gratitude or hope. "Fear is the basest passion of our nature to which motives can be addressed, but it is often the only avenue to the soul."[7]

Cholera had another function besides demonstrating to man the power of the Lord and the futility of earthly values. This was to "promote the cause of righteousness, by sweeping away the obdurate and the incorrigible," and "to drain off the filth and scum which contaminate and defile human society." The great majority of those who fell before this destroyer were the enemies of God. They lived only to scatter about them the "firebrands, arrows, and death" of eternal damna-

[5] Pintard, *Letters from John Pintard to His Daughter Eliza Noel Pintard Davidson, 1816–1833* (New York, 1941), IV, 72, 75, July 13, 19, 1832; *Mercury* (New York), August 1, 1832.

[6] "Subscriber," *Commercial Advertiser* (New York), August 2, 1832.

[7] Gardiner Spring, *A Sermon Preached August 3, 1832, A Day Set Apart in the City of New-York for Public Fasting, Humiliation, and Prayer . . .* (New York, 1832).

tion.[8] The order of the universe required the destruction of
unregenerate sinners on the same ground that human society
required jails and chains for those who disturbed its peace. As
the editor of the *Western Sunday School Messenger* explained
to the "dear children" who studied his weekly column:

Drunkards and filthy, wicked people of all descriptions, are swept
away *in heaps*, as if the Holy God could no longer bear their
wickedness, just as we sweep away a mass of filth when it has
become so corrupt that we cannot bear it. . . . The cholera is not
caused by intemperance and filth, in themselves, but it is a
scourge, a *rod* in the hand of God. . . .[9]

Cholera, the flood, the plague of locusts were temporal means
by which the Lord achieved the world's moral purification.

But there were many other clergymen who could not share
these harsh beliefs, who could not conceive of the God of
Mercy as a vengeful Old Testament war lord, interposing
himself in temporal affairs and punishing the sinner with
death. Only God, they argued, could judge the sins of men,
and none but the self-righteous pharisee would presume to
know his intentions. Did not Christ himself say that those
killed when the tower of Siloam fell were not sinners "above
all men that dwelt in Jerusalem?"[10]

Only miracles could be said to come directly from the hand
of God. "Famine, sword, or pestilence may depopulate a nation, and no link in the thousand stranded chain of causes be
displaced or superseded."[11] Although punishment did not
come directly from the hand of God, such liberal clergymen

[8] *Ibid.*

[9] September 1, 1832.

[10] F. W. P. Greenwood, *Prayer for the Sick. A Sermon Preached at King's Chapel, Boston, on Thursday, August 9, 1832* . . . (Boston, 1832), p. 10. John G. Palfrey, *A Discourse Delivered in the Church in Brattle-Square, Boston, August 9, 1832* . . . (Boston, 1832), p. 10.

[11] Mrs. H. Croswell Tuttle, *History of St. Luke's Church in the City of New York 1820–1920* (New York, 1927), pp. 496–511, reprints a sermon on cholera preached by the Reverend William Whittingham on August 3, 1832, from which this statement is taken.

were quick to add, it was nevertheless a consequence of the actions of men, of their individual and collective sins.

The pestilence was an inevitable result of man's failure to observe the laws of nature. Man has free will, and when he fails to observe these laws, brings inescapable punishment upon himself. Cholera was caused by intemperance and filth and vice—liberals emphasized—conditions which had never been imposed by God.[12] Just as the misuse of a machine must inevitably damage it, so any abuse of our bodies would bring its inescapable punishment.

If one will eat and drink improper substances, or to excess, he . . . must look for disease. . . . We must cease to violate the laws of our constitution—must conform in body and soul to the will of the Creator. . . . It is by this practical obedience that we furnish the best proof of our piety; it is by sacredly observing the laws of our nature, physical, mental, and moral, that we make the most acceptable acknowledgment of Divine Providence, and use the surest means of obtaining for earth the blessings of Heaven.[13]

In the same way as ordinary folk, most religious thinkers managed to keep a foot in both camps, maintaining with traditional rhetoric that cholera was sent by God as a punishment for sin, while at the same time asserting that it did not violate natural laws. All accepted the elaborate doctrine of predisposing causes provided by physicians, a doctrine which seemed to resolve neatly this inherent paradox. The Catholic Bishop of Philadelphia could, for example, warn his diocese that every Christian must realize that cholera was a visitation of God, and in the same pastoral letter, dispense with the Friday fast, since "prudent physicians" regarded fish as an important predisposing cause of the epidemic.[14]

Universalists and their "infidel" allies were quick to point

---

[12] *Gazette and General Advertiser* (New York), July 9, 1832.

[13] Samuel Barrett, *A Sermon Preached in the Twelfth Congregational Church, Boston, Thursday, August 9, 1832 . . .* (Boston, 1832), p. 9. This casual confounding of the spiritual and material was typical of the writings of almost all denominations.

[14] July 12, 1832. *Catholic Telegraph* (Cincinnati) August 4, 1832.

out such seeming inconsistencies. It was "unphilosophical,"
they argued, to consider cholera a direct imposition of the
deity. God operated through "fixed and secondary principles." The day of miracles was past—if it had ever been; every
scientific discovery demonstrated with greater clarity the exclusive power of natural law. Man sees in every natural thing

the effects of uniform laws. . . . In every flower that adorns the
garden, in every blade of grass that adorns the field, and in every
tree that beautifies the grove, he sees the effect of particular laws.
. . . Imperfect as he is, he sees, in the world in which he lives, in
the myriads of worlds around him, one grand, vast, and glorious
system. . . . This glorious world!—this harmonious system! Would
God

> "The dread order break—for whom?—for thee?
> Vile worm! O madness! pride! impiety!"[15]

If man would rid himself of cholera, he must himself "lend a
hand." Natural diseases could only be cured by natural means,
not by the prayer and homilies of the orthodox; one might
with equal logic attempt to convert sinners by cupping, bleeding, and purging. It was always preferable, wrote one physician, to account for natural happenings on "philosophic"
rather than theological principles. "Between Prayer & the answer," jotted another physician in his casebook, "there are
many common place events. No miracle but common human
agencies."[16]

The more perceptive among the orthodox were genuinely
alarmed. God, they feared, was rapidly becoming a prisoner
of his own laws. The intimate and peaceful coexistence with
science enjoyed by most of their brethren must soon culmi-
nate in a religion without a God. Thomas Chalmers, the emi-

[15] "Anti-Formalist," *Philadelphia Liberalist*, August 18, 1832. Such explicitly
deistic rhetoric is not found among the Unitarians or liberal Congregationalists, but only in the writings of the Universalists and freethinkers, infidels
equally in the vocabulary of the orthodox.

[16] Diary of William Darrach, August 20, 1832, Manuscript Division, Pennsylvania Historical Society.

nent Scottish divine, influential in both the United States and the United Kingdom, was intensely aware of such dangers. The most common sort of infidelity, he warned in a widely reprinted fast-day sermon, was that which made the laws of nature autonomous and ignored the overarching power of God. As far as we know, Chalmers conceded, temporal happenings always follow certain laws, certain chains of secondary causes. But man, he affirmed, is capable only of observing the last and crudest of links in this chain. God exerts his influence on a far higher level, one forever hidden from human observation.[17] The danger, of course, lay in the scientist's assumption that he had discovered the meaning of an entire process when he had merely discovered the last in a chain of second causes. We know, a Massachusetts Baptist pointed out to his congregation, that the complex machinery of a mill is powered by gravity which turns the water wheel—but what then is gravity? To state that God had created the world and then allowed it to function independent of his own commands was but an insidious form of infidelity.[18]

It was inevitable that these inconsistent views should clash upon some convenient pretext. And in the outspoken America of Andrew Jackson, such an occasion was not long in presenting itself. It came when President Jackson refused, on constitutional grounds, to recommend a day of public fasting and humiliation. Political animosity in an election year made the conflict even sharper, the Jacksonians holding firmly against any public recommendation of a fast day and their opponents uniformly supporting the idea.

On Monday evening, June 20, a large meeting of New York clergymen and prominent laymen was held at the American Bible Society. Those attending approved unani-

[17] Thomas Chalmers, *The Efficacy of Prayer. A Sermon Preached at St. George's Church, Edinburgh, on Thursday, March 22, 1832, Being the Day Appointed for a National Fast* ... (Boston, 1832).

[18] Elijah Foster, "God's Judgments . . . ," *Christian-Watchman* (Boston), September 14, 1832.

mously a resolution calling for a day of fasting and prayer.[19] Throughout the month of June, such meetings were held in dozens of cities and towns. Episcopal bishops and meetings of the general assemblies and synods of the Presbyterian, Congregational, and Dutch Reformed churches soon appointed fast days for their denominations. City councils, mayors, governors, and eventually Congress received petitions requesting public recommendation of such fast days.

The issue became more than a local one when Henry Clay proposed to the Senate that a joint committee wait upon the President and urge him to appoint a day of national fasting, prayer, and humiliation.[20] This would seem to have been merely a pretext for embarrassing Old Hickory, who had already made public his decision not to recommend a fast day (in a letter to John Schermerhorn, who, as a representative of the General Synod of the Dutch Reformed church, had requested the President to set aside such a day).[21] General Jackson had prudently affirmed his belief in the efficacy of prayer and his hope that America might be protected from the impending pestilence. Nevertheless, he felt that his recommendation of a fast day would be "transcending the limits prescribed by the Constitution for the President." Indeed, he warned, such an action might well interfere with the freedom that religion had always enjoyed in the United States; it was the duty of churches to recommend their own days of religious observance. Two weeks later, Governor Enos Throop of New York replied in a similar vein to a similar request.

These refusals left their authors open to bitter and often personal attacks. Political opponents commented that better

[19] *Evening Post* (New York), June 20, 1832.

[20] There is an account of this episode in Charles Warren, *Odd By-ways in American History* (Cambridge, Mass., 1942), chap. xii, "How Andrew Jackson Opposed a National Fast Day," pp. 221–45.

[21] The letter was dated June 12, 1832, and was reprinted throughout the country before the month was out.

men than Jackson, serving in the same high office, had not entertained such lofty scruples. Washington, Adams, and Madison had all recommended fast days. Talk of the separation of Church and State, they noted with scorn, was that much cant, "the watch word of infidels and drunkards and the very dregs of human society." What man whose "moral sense was not entirely obliterated by sceptical notions" could object to the mere recommendation of a day of fasting? The reasoning in Jackson's letter served to demonstrate the weakness of his intellect, and its motivation to illumine with equal clarity his moral infirmity—his willingness to cater to the sentiments of the lowest order of demagogues and newspapers. But one could expect little else in Jacksonian America, sighed one Connecticut guardian of orthodoxy; the very habits of ungodliness which had made the United States so vulnerable to the disease had also motivated the President in his refusal to proclaim a fast day. The pious and patriotic were proscribed, "while the rabble are courted and applauded, the vicious promoted to office, and the cry which is chanted in their Bacchanalian and nightly revels, is in time of emergency and dread gravely echoed from places of power."[22]

The practical impiety displayed in a refusal to encourage public prayer would, they warned, reap an inevitable punishment. Had not England softened the blow by her day of national prayer? Had not the atheism of France been admonished by the severity of the cholera epidemic in that unhappy country? And certainly America, God's chosen among the nations, was sunk in depravity and had much to repent. Perhaps only cholera, orthodox pulpits warned, was a remedy severe enough to save this once-favored nation from atheism and infidelity. Our political life and our newspapers, the much lauded props of a God-granted democracy, were shamefully polluted; the Sabbath was everywhere flouted—profaned by the movement of stages, steamboats, and even the mails. A

---

[22] "C," *Connecticut Observer* (Hartford), July 16, 1832.

pamphlet distributed by the American Tract Society in enormous quantities—over one hundred and sixty thousand copies in several weeks—summed up the argument: "The highest privileges ever granted to a people have been by multitudes neglected and scorned. Obscene impurities, drunkenness, profaneness, and infidelity, prevail among us to a fearful extent. Iniquity runs down our streets like a river."[23]

Such jeremiads do not seem to have shorn Jackson of many supporters. His followers were accustomed to such gestures of orthodox despair. Orthodox clergymen had thundered against democracy for generations, against Jefferson and Madison as well as against General Jackson. Several denominations, moreover, supported the President in his stand. The Baptists applauded such a clear affirmation of the separation of Church and State. Catholics, Universalists, and Unitarians also approved of Jackson's position. (Only the Universalists, however, carried their opposition to days of public prayer and humiliation to the point of not participating in them, even when such days were set aside by private groups and not local governments.)

Henry Clay was, moreover, ill-chosen as the proponent of national piety. A duelist, drinker, and gambler, the notorious Kentuckian inspired few with faith in his sincerity. The unfortunate Clay had also unwisely remarked in the past that war, famine, and pestilence would be preferable to Andrew Jackson in the White House. He was not allowed to forget that now. Few could have been convinced by his singularly apathetic confession of faith—that he was not a professor of religion, regretted that he was not, and hoped and trusted that he might one day be. "Could he gain votes by it," one Jackson man jeered, "he would kiss the toe of the Pope and prostrate himself before the grand lama."[24]

[23] American Tract Society, *An Appeal on the Subject of the Cholera to the Prepared and Unprepared* (1832), p. 3.

[24] *Times* (Hartford), July 9, August 6, 1832. See also *People's Advocate* (Tolland, Conn.), July 18, 1832.

Though frequently ignored by historians, a peculiarly American variety of anticlericalism had a real place in the rhetoric of Andrew Jackson's democracy.[25] Especially, though not exclusively in New England, the opponents of Old Hickory could be labeled theocrats, as well as Federalists and aristocrats. Orthodox divines had profaned President Madison's fast day with political abuse, Jacksonians charged, and would so profane another if given the opportunity. Even if they refrained from political controversy, the Calvinist priests would pervert a fast day into an occasion for proselytizing. Their "whining cant" would play on the fears of the people, create panic, and only increases the ravages of cholera. The fast-day controversy was an occasion for the expression of long-standing religious and social differences, differences which played a very real part in establishing the political configuration of Jacksonian America.

The self-consciously rationalistic children of the enlightenment, the freethinkers and Universalists, seem to have been almost unanimous in their allegiance to Jackson. Their publications, without exception, ardently supported the General. (Not that all Jacksonians were freethinkers, but all freethinkers were Jacksonians.) At a Tom Paine anniversary, to cite a charming if extreme example, glasses were raised in a toast to "Christianity and the Banks, on their last legs."[26] Of course, most Jacksonians were not infidels. They could, nevertheless, be expected to react vehemently against any proposal that could be branded as a "union of church and state." This principle of separation had, by 1832, become as sacred as the Constitution into which it had been written. Even the most "theocratical" of denominations, Presbyterians, orthodox Congre-

[25] Although using the rhetorical forms of eighteenth-century anticlericalism, Jacksonian anticlericalism was directed not against the Catholic church, which played no significant part in American life, but against the domestic theocrats, especially the Presbyterians and orthodox Congregationalists.

[26] Albert Post, *Popular Freethought in America, 1825–1850* (New York, 1943), p. 157.

gationalists, and Roman Catholics, made regular obeisances in its direction.[27]

Talk of fast days and divine mercy was merely part of a clerical plot to effect the union of Church and State. So at least the radicals charged; pious wailings over cholera were but one link in the chain of bigotry and superstition which the orthodox would fasten upon the American people.

> The skilled in lore and mystery
> From time to time await,
> Nor slip one opportunity,
> *To marry Church and State!*
> Hope gives them dreams of wealth and ease,
> And Beelzebub sends pride,
> And whilst they sleep, *the sheaves leap up,*
> *And on the tithe cart ride!*
> Reflect—ye who drink deep at doubt's
> Broad fountain—full and free;
> Can priests avert the shafts of fate,
> or change our destiny?[28]

George Henry Evans, the radical journalist, urged his readers to ignore a fast-day recommendation made by New York City's Common Council. Such a recommendation constituted an "insidious and dangerous encroachment" upon the separation of Church and State. It would be observed by "none but the ignorant bigot, and the less ignorant enemy of freedom of opinion."[29]

Actually, Jackson and Throop were not typical in their actions. Executive appointment of days of fasting and prayer was accepted procedure, especially in New England. The governors of at least eleven states eventually proclaimed fast

[27] John R. Bodo, *The Protestant Clergy and Public Issues, 1812–1848* (Princeton, 1954), asserts that such theoretical respect for the separation of Church and State did not impede orthodox attempts to make American government "Christian." Catholic papers were, of course, fervent in their praise of this principle of government.

[28] *Sentinel* (New York), June 30, 1832.

[29] *Sentinel* (New York), July 31, 1832.

days in an effort to avert cholera.[30] Yet most, wary of the issue of Church and State, were careful to state that their proclamations were merely recommendations and not executive decrees.

No one, regardless of his theoretical position, could remain idle while the sinner perished. Men who believed cholera to be a God-sent scourge espoused exactly the same prophylactic measures as those who attributed the prevalence of the disease to the injustice of human society.[31] Common humanity allied with primal fear demanded that prompt and effective action be taken.

An integral part of a faith in the Lord was faith in the efficacy of his means. Clergymen of all denominations agreed that prayer alone could not prevent cholera. It would be as much an abuse of the power of prayer to expect it to avert cholera while streets remained filthy as for the husbandman to anticipate a harvest where he had planted no seed. If science could discover laws by which cholera might be prevented, religion itself would prompt us to observe them. What, indeed, were medicines but treasures drawn from God's great storehouse?

So far from despising them, therefore, the religious man will regard them as things divine; he will regard medical skill, as an art and gift divine; and he will make use of them when necessary. . . .

[30] These included Connecticut, Georgia, Indiana, Kentucky, Maryland, Massachusetts, New Jersey, North Carolina, Ohio, Pennsylvania, and Vermont. In Rhode Island, the legislature proclaimed a fast day.

[31] The dictates of Christian Science would have been regarded as not only absurd but impious—this despite a current view that nineteenth-century clergymen opposed the prevention of disease as irreverence; cf. Reginald Reynolds, *Cleanliness and Godliness* . . . (Garden City, 1946), pp. 116–17. David Schneider, in *History of Public Welfare in the State of New York 1609–1866* (Chicago, 1938), p. 256, wrote of the New York cholera epidemic of 1832 that "many individuals, including physicians doubted whether any positive measures to check an epidemic should be taken at all, on the ground that a plague was a God sent form of punishment. . . ." No evidence is cited to support this statement, and I have not found any which would.

He is not a fatalist. He believes it to be disobedience to God, not to employ the aids which God furnishes for his use. . . .[32]

Common prudence as well demanded that the epidemic be fought as effectively as possible. The reassurance garnered from the doctrine of predisposing causes, and from belief in the non-contagiousness of the disease, was vitiated by the conviction that cholera could become indiscriminately virulent if it were to rage uncontrolled in particularly dirty and confined locations. (And what city did not have its own "Five Points"?) The "epidemic influence" generated under such circumstances might well prove fatal even to those of regular habits; the "moral fens and morasses" of society were potential sources of danger to every member of the community.

[32] F. W. P. Greenwood, *op. cit.,* pp. 12–13.

III. OR MAN'S INJUSTICE?

Asiatic cholera was a disease not only of the sinner but of the poor. Neither poverty nor wealth seemed to be an accidental condition, and many well-to-do Americans saw in their riches visible testimony to the regularity of their habits. The vices—intemperance, immorality, impiety—which doomed a man to poverty were the same ones which predisposed him to cholera. The Irish and Negroes, the most filthy, intemperate, and imprudent portion of the population and hence the poorest of Americans, were, not surprisingly, the most frequent victims of cholera.

Americans fearful of cholera in the spring of 1832 were encouraged by the reflection that there was little real poverty in the United States. "People call themselves poor among us," Americans confidently reflected, "who never knew, from birth to death, what it is to lack a wholesome meal, or comfortable clothing, or clean and good lodgings." The American mechanic had qualities far superior to those of his European counterpart. In "true worth and usefulness," he was "scarcely surpassed" by even the farmer. Wealth was, moreover, no hereditary perquisite. It seemed to lie within each man's grasp: "The sons of the poor die rich—while the sons of the rich die poor."[1] The vices which predisposed to cholera were charac-

[1] *Gazette* (Salem), n.d., cited in the *National Gazette* (Philadelphia), August 7, 1832; *Free Press* (Detroit), July 18, 1832.

teristic in Europe of both the very highest and the very lowest classes. America, which had few of either, seemed to have little to fear. "The middle and respectable ranks," to which the great mass of Americans belonged, were the "most sober and temperate" of classes, and would, accordingly, escape though both high and low be swept away.[2] Unfortunately, not all of the poor were hard-working mechanics, farmers, or shopkeepers.

Though there existed a poverty so exalted as to form a Christian virtue, there was, Americans believed, "another and more frequent kind of poverty which is both the consequence and origin of vice." Idleness and intemperance were not only vices often found among the poor; they were, in the minds of many Americans, the chief cause of their poverty. Such habits, moreover, not only clothed men in rags, but were "the natural parent of disease."[3] It was not the healthy and industrious workingman who need fear cholera but the vicious and indolent among the poor.

Cholera seemed indeed to be a "poor man's plague." In Paris, there were so few deaths outside of the lower classes, that the poor regarded the epidemic as a poison plot fomented by the aristocracy and executed by the doctors. The majority of the 853 cholera victims in Baltimore in the summer of 1832 were of the "most worthless" sort. In contrast, of the 362 subscribers to Quebec's Exchange Coffee House, all persons "enjoying comfortable and good circumstances, only one died." Even if the epidemic did eventually spread to the better sort, it always began among the lowest and most dissolute. To suf-

[2] *Yeoman's Gazette* (Concord, Mass.), July 7, 1832; *Workingman's Shield* (Cincinnati), I (September 8, 1832), 15. Workers with their hands, the artisan and the mechanic, it was argued, would find an additional measure of safety in the strength of their work-hardened constitutions.

[3] Marshall Tufts, *A History of the Cholera*, pp. 59–60; "B," *Observer* (New York), July 21, 1832; *Thomsonian Recorder*, I (1832), 63; John Bell and D. Francis Condie, *All the Material Facts in the History of Epidemic Cholera* (Philadelphia, 1832), p. 47. This ambivalent and contradictory attitude toward the poor continued throughout the century, the negative aspects increasing as confidence in America's divine exemption from European strife and misery waned. See John Hay's *Breadwinners*, for example.

fer from cholera was socially inexcusable. One New York physician failed for some time to report a case in a young lady "of tender constitution." He feared that "the circumstances of her being noticed in the papers, as Cholera, would produce a mental depression detrimental to her final recovery." "Confined mostly to the lower classes," cholera was, in the words of an irreverent young medical student, "decidedly vulgar."[4]

The disease did, in reality, select a disproportionately large number of its victims from among the poor, a fact verified in almost every cholera epidemic for which statistics are available. In Hamburg, the case rate in 1892 among those with an income of a thousand marks or less was nineteen times greater than the rate among those with an income of fifty thousand marks or more. In New York during the epidemic in 1832, almost all who died were buried either at the Potter's Field or in St. Patrick's cemetery. Of one hundred cholera deaths on one July day, ninety-five were buried in the Potter's Field. In Richmond, Virginia, the poorhouse graveyard was the last resting place for nine-tenths of those who had died of cholera.[5]

The real suffering of the poor is easily explained. They lived in the worst houses in the most crowded portions of the city and could not afford to flee when threatened by the epidemic. In New York, for example, it was not until death and public removal had thinned their ranks that the epidemic began to subside. Basement apartments were from four to six feet below the surface of the ground, and from these warrens came the "greater proportions and worst forms of cases."[6]

---

[4] Dr. J. C. Lovel to the Board of Health, July 12, 1832, Filed Papers of the Common Council, File Drawer T-592, Municipal Archives and Records Center; Henry Lincoln to May Ann Lincoln, August 12, 1832, Lincoln Family Papers, in the possession of Mrs. J. F. Townsend, New Haven, Connecticut.

[5] Bernhard J. Stern, *Society and Medical Progress* (Princeton, 1941), p. 134; Report of the Potter's Field Keeper, Cornelius Myers, to the Board of Health, City Clerk's Papers, U-57, Municipal Archives and Records Center; *Constitutional Whig* (Richmond), October 9, 1832.

[6] N.Y.C. Board of Health, *Reports of Hospital Physicians* . . . (New York, 1832), pp. 14–15.

Unable to afford water brought from outside the city, the poor had to depend upon the river or New York's shallow and polluted wells for their supply.

To many Americans, the extent of poverty revealed by the epidemic was genuinely disturbing. Only on such extraordinary occasions, wrote one New York matron, was the "dreadful misery and distress of the City known." A Cincinnati editor observed that if the disease was caused by poor food, poor lodgings, filth, and intemperance, "the number of victims gives us a melancholy idea of the present state of society." Physicians, many of whom were making calls in unaccustomed quarters, were acutely conscious of the misery in which so many of their fellow citizens existed. A Lexington, Kentucky, practitioner was amazed at the amount of "squalid wretchedness" revealed by the cholera epidemic in the midst of what he had assumed to be general prosperity. Shocked by the conditions of the Irish workingmen in London, a young Boston physician wrote home arguing that the only way to check the epidemic was to remove "the *predisposition of the poor.* . . . Give food to the hungry, clothe the naked, remove the filth from the habitations of the poor, and the cholera will quickly disappear."[7]

To a professed radical like George Henry Evans, cholera was no heavenly decree, but rather an inevitable result of human injustice; men, not God, permitted filth, wretchedness, and poverty to exist. Evans advocated a graduated income tax to provide the funds necessary to make the recurrence of *any* disease impossible. For he believed that the origin and spread of cholera, and of disease in general, was due to "*poverty, occasioned by unjust remuneration of labor.*"[8] Though not a

[7] Mrs. P. Roosevelt to S. R. Johnson, July 13, 1832, Roosevelt Papers, General Theological Seminary; *Cincinnati Mirror*, I (August 18, 1832), 191; Lunsford P. Yandell, "An Account of the Spasmodic Cholera, as It Appeared in the City of Lexington, in June 1833," *Transylvania Journal of Medicine*, VI (1833), 202–3; Forbes Winslow, *Medical Magazine*, I (1832), 261–62.

[8] *Workingman's Advocate* (New York), August 11, 1832.

scourge of the vicious, cholera had taught a lesson—a very simple one: there must be an end to poverty, destitution, and ignorance.

> Yet still will wealth presumptuous cry
> What though the hand of death be thus outstretched
> It will not reach the lordly and the high
> But only strike the lowly and the wretched,
> Tush!—what have we to quail at? Let us fold
> Our arms, and trust to luxury and gold.
>
> O thou reforming cholera! thou'rt sent
> Not as a scourge alone, but as a teacher. . . .[9]

To at least some Americans, cholera seemed an unmistakable indictment of the society which allowed it to exist. Cholera was but a most recent and acute consequence of man's chronic inhumanity to man.[10]

Who were the worst sufferers? There was no doubt in the minds of most observers; the Irish and Negroes seemed its foreordained victims. Easily panic-stricken, filthy, intemperate, and imprudent, they offered little resistance to the onslaughts of the disease.

Despite rumors that Negroes in Canada had escaped unscathed, it was soon apparent that they suffered as much as the most ill-favored of the white population.[11] In Philadelphia, the

---

[9] "The Cholera Morbus," *Atlas*, IV (1831–32), 109.

[10] Boston Board of Health Commissioners, *Report of the Medical Deputation Appointed . . . To Visit New York . . .* (Boston, 1832), p. 3, strongly affirms that the idea that the disease affects classes differently "is true only in reference to habits, and not to condition. The laboring part of the community, when temperate and prudent in their modes of living, are as likely as any who could be named, to escape the disease."

[11] As a number of contemporaries pointed out, this false belief probably had its origin in the fact that there were almost no Negroes in Quebec or Montreal. See the *Commercial Advertiser* (New York), July 21, 1832, and the *Cholera Gazette*, August 1, 1832, for reports contradicting this rumor. Only one physician, but that the ordinarily astute clinician Daniel Drake, felt that the Negro had any racial affinity for the disease. Drake, *An Account of the Epidemic Cholera, as It Appeared in Cincinnati* (New York, 1832), p. 19.

case rate among Negroes was almost twice as great as that among whites—probably a reliable, if informal, index to the poverty in which the North's free Negroes lived.[12] Whether he was free or slave, Americans believed, the Negro's innate character invited cholera. He was, with few exceptions, filthy and careless in his personal habits, lazy and ignorant by temperament. A natural fatalist, moreover, he took no steps to protect himself from disease and shared, to an exaggerated extent, the distaste of the poor for hospitals and the medical profession. "Thoughtless and careless," the free Negro had few resources beyond the product of his daily labor, and would not work at all, most Americans were convinced, unless threatened by starvation. Accordingly, the freedman enjoyed a ward's status even after manumission. In Lynchburg, for example, free Negroes failing to comply with sanitary regulations received ten lashes on the bare back. No punishments were contemplated for white offenders. As a final item in the sum of their misery, Negroes were the defenseless subjects for the experiments of eager southern physicians. One such practitioner, hearing that cholera impaired "nervous sensibility," poured boiling water on the legs of a Negro man already comatose, "which he felt so acutely, that he leaped up instantly and appeared to be in great agony."[13]

Throughout the summer of 1832, editors of southern newspapers filled their columns with recipes and hygienic recommendations, while physicians published numbers of cholera treatises specifically for worried planters. (Though the hygienic recommendations were, in many cases, quite sensible, the ingredients of the recipes which accompanied them must certainly have put an abrupt end to the lives of many bondsmen.) Richmond, anticipating cholera, established special hos-

[12] Samuel Jackson, "Personal Observations and Experience of Epidemic or Malignant Cholera in the City of Philadelphia," *American Journal of the Medical Sciences*, XI (1832), 293.

[13] P. M. Kollock, "An Account of Cholera, as It Prevailed in the City of Savannah . . . ," *Southern Medical Journal*, I (1836), 329–30.

pitals for the Negro workers in her tobacco factories. Many masters—like Henry Clay who postponed a political trip rather than leave Ashland and his "family" of sixty when they were threatened by the epidemic—felt deep concern for the welfare of their "people."[14]

Judging, however, from the tone of hundreds of southern articles on cholera, it was to the pocket and not the heart that such cautionary appeals had to be made. The "cry of fanaticism, colonization, abolition," wrote one Virginia physician, greeted any proposal for ameliorating the condition of the slaves. Cholera was but the final proof, he continued, of the "deformity and gross stupidity" of the Old Dominion's labor system.

A quarter plantation well supplied with all the necessary labour &c., given up by its owner to exclusive controul of one of your thorough fellows, whose interest is made to depend entirely on the amount produced each year, furnishes to my mind a picture of moral deformity, the most frightful, and the most loathesome in the *world*. Upon such estates so situated, I expect to hear every day of the occurrence of cholera. . . .[15]

And the progress of cholera through the South was clear enough proof that where Negroes lived best, they lived longest and suffered least. Perhaps, wrote a Louisiana plantation mistress, avarice might produce the improvement in their conditions which humanity had never been able to achieve.[16]

The newly arrived immigrants played an equally tragic role during the epidemic; populating the foulest slums of America's cities, they suffered far out of proportion to their numbers. To most respectable Americans, however, their premature deaths were the inevitable consequence of a life mis-

---

[14] *Enquirer* (Richmond), August 17, September 18, 1832; Henry Clay to Peter B. Porter, July 2, 1833, Peter B. Porter Papers, Buffalo Historical Society.

[15] "A Country Physician," *Enquirer* (Richmond), October 2, 1832.

[16] Mary Holley to her daughter, November 25, 1832, Division of Archives, University of Texas, cited in William D. Postell, *The Health of Slaves* (Baton Rouge, 1951), p. 78.

spent. In New York, the Board of Health reported that "the low Irish suffered the most, being exceedingly dirty in their habits, much addicted to intemperance and crowded together into the worst portions of the city."[17] Even in rural areas, Irish workers on canals and railroads were often the first and sometimes the only ones to suffer from cholera. If fortunate enough to escape with his life, the immigrant still had to bear the onus of having brought the disease with him on his passage to the New World. Despite the assurances of medical men that cholera was not contagious, the newly arrived immigrant found all doors closed to him. Hundreds wandered starved and half-naked along the Canadian border.

The cholera epidemic was, to many Americans, but one of the alarming consequences of an unprecedented increase in immigration. Even the optimistic Hezekiah Niles felt that such quantities of labor would only add to the difficulties of native workers in finding employment. Our cities, the Baltimore editor accused, had long been taxed "for the support of miserable foreigners, just arrived. Our poor houses are filled with them. Let not those who have sucked the orange throw its skin at us."[18] Mrs. Peter Roosevelt predicted that the entire nation would soon be "overrun with paupers," for the immigrants were, with few exceptions, "a set of beggars."[19] The Irish had already earned themselves the resentment of the godly for the skill and rapidity with which they had filled the roles of politico and saloonkeeper. And few Americans were willing to deny that the liquor trade and corrupt municipal governments had multiplied the number of cholera victims.

Americans believed that theirs was a nation in which abso-

[17] N.Y.C. Board of Health, *Reports of Hospital Physicians* . . . (New York, 1832), pp. 14–15.

[18] *Niles' Register*, XLII (July 21, 1832), 372; Niles reserved most of his dislike for the Irish. He exempted the Germans, "an industrious and moral race," from his strictures and rejoiced that America was still a haven for the oppressed. *Ibid.*, XLIII (September 29, 1832), 68.

[19] Mrs. P. Roosevelt to S. R. Johnson, July 13, 1832, Roosevelt Papers, General Theological Seminary.

lute freedom reigned; the people governed, and continued high standards of education and morality were necessary if democracy was to survive. Yet all too often, the foreigners pouring in upon the United States had notions either despotic and monarchic or else vicious and licentious. Philip Hone, the diarist, self-made man, and eminently conservative New Yorker, could find little encouraging in the arrival of such immigrants. "They have brought the cholera this year," he observed in September,

and they will always bring wretchedness and want. The boast that our country is the asylum for the oppressed in other parts of the world is very philanthropic and sentimental, but I fear that we shall before long derive little comfort from being made the almshouse and refuge for the poor of other countries.[20]

Despite the immigrant's often distasteful personal characteristics, the great majority of native Americans still regarded him as more deserving of pity than censure. He had fled centuries of poverty and oppression to the one land which offered him liberty and asylum; cholera was but a final entry in the sum of his misfortunes. Having survived the hardships of a debilitating ocean voyage, he must now wander hungry and ill-clothed because Americans feared that he might be a carrier of disease. Throughout the eastern United States, the benevolent contributed to the relief of these homeless wayfarers.

Even Roman Catholics benefited from a tolerance far greater than that accorded them later in the century. Though admittedly ignorant and superstitious, they received little but praise for their conduct during the epidemic. (Those opposed to the "puritan priests" found particular enjoyment in praising Roman Catholic benevolence.) If anything, the heroic works of the Catholic clergy and religious women during the epidemic acted, if only momentarily, to moderate an already

<hr>

[20] Diary of Philip Hone, September 20, 1832, Manuscript Division, New York Historical Society.

waxing temper of anti-Catholicism.[21] Even so militant a Protestant as Ezra Stiles Ely, editor of the ultra-orthodox *Philadelphian* and founder of the Christian Party a few years before, had to admit that the Catholic clergy had shown great fidelity. In a half-dozen cities, the Sisters of Charity nursed the sick when other nurses could not be found. This "practical tendency" in their benevolence, allied with a romantically tinged view of the sisters as self-sacrificing women, could not but produce sympathy for the church to which they had dedicated their lives.[22] The fidelity of all ranks among the Catholic clergy was doubly striking when contrasted with the frequent defections among their Protestant contemporaries. Many ministers chose to take their summer vacations during cholera epidemics, while others were accused of barricading themselves in their houses and refusing to answer the calls of the sick. As Catholics were quick to point out, the poor, unless Catholic, were left without spiritual guidance during a time of mortal and spiritual peril. "The poor of no other church have a clergy, it is only the rich."[23]

[21] This is also suggested by Hugh Nolan in his biography of *The Most Reverend Francis Patrick Kenrick, Third Bishop of Philadelphia, 1830–1851* (Philadelphia, 1948), p. 159.

[22] *Philadelphian*, August 30, 1832. For additional comment on the Sisters of Charity, see *Beacon* (St. Louis), November 15, 1832; *Illinois Whig* (Vandalia), November 28, 1832; *Franklin Repository* (Chambersburg, Pa.), August 21, 1832; *Patriot* (Baltimore), n.d., cited in the *United States Telegraph* (Washington, D.C.), August 17, 1832; *Niles' Register*, XLII (August 18, 1832), 439; *Ulster Palladium* (Kingston, N.Y.), August 29, 1832; *Liberalist* (Philadelphia), September 15, 1832.

[23] *United States Catholic Intelligencer*, March 23, July 27, August 17, September 21, 1832. John Pintard was forced to comment that "whatever be the errors of Roman Catholics, we must give them credit for their zeal & faith. God help us Protestants, I wish that we manifested more of both. . . ." *Letters from John Pintard to His Daughter Eliza Noel Pintard Davidson, 1816–1833* (New York, 1941), IV, 92.

IV. THE MEDICAL PROFESSION I

American medicine was provincial. The average physician, ill-paid and poorly trained, struggled constantly to retain the dignity and prestige traditionally accorded his learned profession. The cholera epidemic of 1832 was an unavoidable challenge to his status and, perhaps more importantly, to his ideas and assumptions.

Cholera was a manageable disease. Of this the regular physicians were assured. It could be deprived of its malignancy if the "premonitory symptoms" were treated in time; and it had been proven that a "painless diarrhea" was the universal premonitory symptom. Belief in the efficacy of this—or some—principle of treatment was a necessary and, perhaps, inevitable means by which physicians and laymen alike preserved their equanimity when surrounded by uncertainty and death. "All that was obscure, mysterious, and empirical" had been replaced by a cure "dependent on rules of science easily comprehended."[1] Only those who had first predisposed themselves, and had then ignored the premonitory symptoms, became cholera victims. In dozens of American communities, physicians could confidently point to cases of incipient cholera that had been cured by opportune treatment.[2]

[1] James B. Kirk, *Practical Observations on Cholera Asphyxia* . . . (New York, 1832), p. 4.

[2] These encouraging results were almost certainly due to the fact that they were treating persons who did not have cholera, or who had at the very worst a minor case.

Still, there were problems of therapy. How was the preliminary painless diarrhea to be treated? And what was to be done
for those unfortunates who had progressed beyond the premonitory symptoms? Here it seemed that no two physicians
could agree precisely, each practitioner employing a favorite
remedy or combination of remedies. A representative course
of treatment was that recommended by New York's Special
Medical Council. They advised general bloodletting "to mitigate the spasms and render the system more susceptible to the
action of the grand remedy, Mercury." The patient's skin
was to be kept warm by continued rubbing with such substances as powdered chalk, cayenne pepper, mercury oint-
ment, and calomel; he could be regarded as out of danger
"when [his] mouth becomes sore or the discharges bilious,
from the operation of mercury."[3]

Calomel, a chalky mercury compound, employed almost
universally as a cathartic, was the most widely used cholera
remedy. Immense dosages were prescribed: quantities of the
drug which a generation before had been thought "fit for a
horse" were now used routinely for children. The suppurat-
ing gums symptomatic of mercury poisoning were regarded
by many physicians as a hopeful sign, an indication that the
drug was working efficiently. Other physicians relied on
massive doses of laudanum or bleeding. The more eclectic
combined all three—laudanum, calomel, and bleeding.[4] A
Louisiana physician boasted that he had drawn "blood enough
to float the General Jackson steamboat, and gave calomel
enough to freight her."[5]

This was conservative treatment. The more radical advo-

[3] N.Y.C. Board of Health, *Questions of the Board of Health, in relation to
the Malignant Cholera, with the Answers of the Special Medical Council*
(New York, 1832), p. 5.

[4] "Calomel in Cholera," *Medical Magazine*, II (1833–34), 596; John Esten
Cooke, "Remarks on Spasmodic Cholera," *Transylvania Journal of Medicine*,
V (1832), 498–99; *Ibid.*, VI (1833), 207, 331, 553.

[5] Charles A. Lee, *Boston Medical and Surgical Journal*, VII (August 15,
1832), 18.

cated such expedients as tobacco smoke enemas, electric shocks, and the injection of saline solutions into the veins. The president of New York State Medical Society, a practical soul, suggested that the rectum be plugged with beeswax or oilcloth so as to check the diarrhea. Charles G. Finney must have been only one among many to recall that the means used to cure him of cholera left his "system" with a "terrible shock, from which it took long to recover."[6]

Few physicians were able to admit, even to themselves, that they could do nothing for a well-developed case of cholera. Only a man as candid and as perceptive as Sir Thomas Watson, the great English clinician, could have concluded, that "if the balance could be fairly struck, and the exact truth ascertained, I question whether we should find the aggregate mortality from cholera, in this country, was any way disturbed by our craft."[7]

There were never enough physicians to treat every case of cholera. Quacks of every description flourished, encouraged not only by the scarcity but by the high fees and draconic remedies of the "regulars." Many common folk were ministered to by kind-hearted neighbors, relatives, or even clergymen. Others dosed themselves with the cures and preventives

---

[6] For tobacco as a remedy, see J. N. Casanova, *General Observations Respecting Cholera Morbus* (Philadelphia and Baltimore, 1832), pp. 61–65; the president of the state medical society was Thomas Spencer, *Practical Observations on Epidemic Diarrhoea, Known as the Epidemic Cholera . . .* (Utica, 1832); Finney, *Memoirs of Rev. Charles G. Finney* (New York, 1876), pp. 320–21. Though the injection of saline solutions seems to us reasonable, the manner in which it was undertaken tended to discredit it and, by implication, the physiological reasoning upon which this therapy was based. (European physicians had, by comparing the proportion of "liquids" and "solids" in the blood of normal persons with that found in cholera sufferers, found a much higher proportion of solids in the blood of those afflicted with cholera—hence, the recommendation of saline solutions to restore a proper balance.)

[7] Watson, *Lectures on the Principles and Practice of Physic . . .* (Philadelphia, 1844), p. 722. At least a few American physicians had begun to reach similar conclusions. Cf. George C. Shattuck, Jr., to G. C. Shattuck, September 10, 1832, Shattuck Papers, Manuscript Division, Massachusetts Historical Society; Drs. Alwyn Bogard, J. F. D. Lobstein, and W. Anderson to the Board of Health, August 16, 1832, Filed Papers of the Common Council, File Drawer T-590, Municipal Archives and Records Center.

advertised everywhere in newspapers and handbills. A Philadelphia handbill proclaimed a nostrum for "the Prevention
and Cure of Cholera Morbus, and *all other diseases.*" Were
this medicine generally used, the advertisement emphatically
concluded, "death from *any* kind of disease, would be a *rare*
occurrence." In the absence of physicians, necessity often dictated therapeutics. The Mormons, for instance, treated their
sick by immersing them in icy water, "which had the desired
effect of stopping the purging, vomiting, and cramping."[8]

The conflicting and uniformly unsuccessful modes of treatment followed by the medical profession shook an already
insecure public confidence. Some of the poor and unen-
lightened hid their symptoms as long as they could, unwilling
to trust themselves to a physician's care, while even the most
credulous displayed an increasing skepticism toward the
therapeutic claims of the profession.

Alas! then for the public, for whom doctors and cholera are con-
tending; they watch the fierce onslaught, and ever and anon are
struck by the random blows that proceed from the combatants.
Yes! for "Cholera kills, and Doctors slay, and every foe will have
its way!"[9]

The old adage that "doctors will differ" was never better
exemplified than now, when there was greatest need for
unanimity, bitterly observed William Cullen Bryant's New
York *Evening Post* (July 9). But the doctors themselves were
at sea. What, wailed one physician, were we "small fry" to do,
when there was no "paramount authority," whose opinions
might safely be quoted?

The behavior of many physicians during the epidemic did
little to increase the prestige of their profession. In some cases,
panic-stricken physicians fled from the epidemic, while others
were charged with profiteering. Night calls were particularly

[8] The handbill was reprinted in the *Journal of Health,* III (1832), 332–33;
Heber C. Kimball, "Journal," *Times and Seasons* (Nauvoo, Ill.), VI (March
15, 1845), 840.

[9] *Cholera Bulletin,* July 23, 1832.

onerous, and many physicians would not make them under any circumstances. Some, victims of a public unwillingness to admit the presence of cholera, were accused of manufacturing cases in order to further their own reputations. And, despite their generally circumspect attitude toward accepted morality, "materialistic" physicians were persistently attacked by temperance advocates for prescribing port and brandy in the treatment of the disease.

Still, to most practitioners, the epidemic meant long hours of exhausting, discouraging, and dangerous work. And, in the main, physicians fulfilled their duties in good faith. For each complaint that doctors had fled, there was at least one hymn of praise for their fidelity. In New York, at least ten physicians were cholera victims. (Each of the ten medical men of the city's Second Ward was presented with a piece of silver, "suitably inscribed," for his gratuitous services to the poor during the epidemic.) It took courage to be a physician in such times, a simple truth recognized in the higher fees which were, by custom, charged during an epidemic.[10]

To their credit as well, American physicians seem eagerly to have sought understanding of this new disease. Medical journals were filled with the writings of Frenchmen, Englishmen, Germans, and Russians on the nature and treatment of cholera, while dozens of American medical men traveled to Canada or New York to study the disease. Others wrote to colleagues and teachers who had treated cholera, begging their advice.[11] Many were of an inquiring disposition and did

[10] New York City Board of Health, Minutes, December 22, 1832, Municipal Archives and Records Center; George Rosen, Fees and Fee Bills: Some Economic Aspects of Medical Practice in Nineteenth-Century America (Supplement of the Bulletin of the History of Medicine, No. 6, 1946).

[11] In surveying local newspapers, I have found mention of at least twenty-three physicians who traveled to New York to observe the disease. They came from points as distant as Lynchburg, Virginia, and Gardiner, Maine. Some were reimbursed by local health boards, others by "associations of citizens," while still others paid their own way. The College of Physicians of Philadelphia possesses a bound scrapbook filled with letters written by former students to Professor Samuel Jackson in the summer of 1832, asking guidance in the treatment of this exotic disease.

not limit themselves to collecting second-hand information. They performed dozens of autopsies—regarded as dangerous even by men who denied the contagiousness of the disease.

No physician showed more courage and integrity during the epidemic than did Daniel Drake, the Benjamin Rush of America's West. Defying the abuse of his fellow Cincinnatians, he had been the first in the city to announce that cholera had broken out. Later, he denied that cholera claimed as victims only the vicious and poverty-stricken; drunkards, he felt himself compelled to conclude, were no more liable to attacks of the disease than the temperate. "I expect," he wrote,

to be censured for publishing this fact. But I am writing a medical history, not a temperance address . . . the cause of scientific truth suffers from the suppression not less than the perversion of facts. There are obligations to science, as well as morality; and they can never, in fact, be incompatible.[12]

Despite its often heroic exertions, the medical profession could ill-afford the burden of its own pretensions. A pragmatic society found little in their results to justify claims to a monopoly of medical practice. His own attainments, many Americans believed, rather than legislative fiat, should determine the physician's status. It was a poor compliment to the "intelligence and discernment of the population," to assume that they were incompetent to choose their own physicians.

There were many who made a profession of medicine without benefit of license or diploma. The most numerous and vocal of these were the followers of Thomsonianism. A homegrown medical heresy, Thomsonianism, or botanic medicine, rejected drugs of mineral origin, relying on the "natural" powers of certain herbs.[13] The basic mixtures were patented

[12] Drake, *An Account of the Epidemic Cholera, as It Appeared in Cincinnati* (New York, 1832), pp. 18–19.

[13] Why minerals were less natural than herbs is not clear, though the idea is appealing, as can be seen in the long life of such statements, which have

and could be purchased in kits for home use. Do-it-yourself medicine appealed to Jacksonian America.

There was no place in the United States for a privileged and monopolistic class of physicians. Thomsonian attacks identified the regulars with monopoly, traditionalism, and intolerance. Like priest-craft, doctor-craft would soon be put to an end. "May the time soon come when men and women will become their own priests, physicians and lawyers—when self-government, equal rights and moral philosophy will take the place of all popular crafts of every description."[14] Samuel Thomson, founder of botanic medicine and something of a versifier, summed up the argument against the status-conscious learned professions.

> The nest of college-birds are three,
> *Law, Physic and Divinity;*
> And while these three remain combined,
> They keep the world oppressed and blind.
> On Lab'rers money lawyers feast,
> Also the Doctor and the Priest;
>
> . . . .
>
> The *Priest* pretends to save the soul,
> Doctors to make the body whole;
> For money, lawyers make their plea;
> We'll save it and dismiss the three.
>
> . . . .
>
> Come freemen all, unveil your eyes,
> If you this slavish yoke despise;
> Now is the time to be set free,
> From Priests' and Doctors' slavery.[15]

persisted until the present time. An excellent account of the botanic system is that by Alex Berman, "The Impact of the Nineteenth-Century Botanico-Medical Movement in American Pharmacy and Medicine" (unpublished doctoral dissertation, University of Wisconsin, 1954).

[14] "R. H.," *Thomsonian Recorder*, I (1832), 89.

[15] Samuel Thomson, *Learned Quackery Exposed: Or Theory According to Art* . . . (Boston, 1836), pp. 17–19. See also *Thomsonian Recorder*, I (1832), vii; John Thomson, *A Philosophical Theory of an "Empiric," Proved Practically* . . . (Albany, 1833), p. 5.

Only the dullard would pay the doctor, the priest, or the lawyer to do his thinking for him. Where was the practical justification for the proscriptive demands of the learned professions? The lesson of cholera was clear enough: those physicians who had not fled had merely hurried the passage of their patients from this world.

Thomsonianism was a rural and lower-class phenomenon. In New York, for instance, Thomsonian petitions to the Board of Health were crudely scrawled on cheap paper. Equalitarian, antiauthoritarian, and anticlerical, the rhetoric of Thomsonianism was as peculiarly a product of Jacksonian America as the image of Old Hickory himself—of whom, one assumes, the devotees of botanic medicine were almost unanimous supporters. (It is tempting to visualize the great-grandson of a Thomsonian healer with a set of *Appeal to Reason* or Ingersoll's speeches on the same shelf which had borne his great-grandfather's cabinet of herbs, tinctures, and infusions.)

Spokesmen for the regular medical corps were quite conscious that the attack made upon their status was only part of a thoroughgoing assault which menaced all of the learned professions. In the words of one physician arguing against the incorporation of a botanic medical society in New York, the prosperity of the medical profession was

inseparable from the prosperity of every well-regulated community. If it fall, the other liberal professions will be weakened in their character, impaired in their usefulness, and finally they will all sink into mere trades, for the cunning, the avaricious, and the unprincipled.[16]

Fortunately, the medical profession still retained the patronage of the wealthy, the educated, and the respectable.

Though physicians could not agree on a means of treating cholera, their opinions of the predisposing causes and of the proper means of prophylaxis were almost unanimous. Poor and marshy land was dangerous, as were filthy and ill-venti-

[16] *Transactions of the Medical Society of the State of New York*, 1832–33, p. 84, appendix.

lated apartments. The poor who lived in such squalor were to be removed to clean, dry, and airy houses as soon as possible. Even more important was a careful attention to diet; not only strong drink but every kind of food not easily digestible had to be avoided scrupulously. Newspapers printed scores of stories of temperate men who had died as a result of eating a green apple or chewing a plug of tobacco. Fear was another potent predisposing cause—fear or any other violent emotion.

In 1832, the idea that disease was a specific, well-defined biological entity was controversial and, indeed, highly suspect. Many American physicians were careful to disclaim any belief in what they termed "ontology." ("That is, in the idea that disease is an *entity*—a being—a something added to the system."[17]) Disease was a protean and dynamic condition. Psychic and somatic ills were not rigidly demarcated: mental, moral, climatic, and hygienic factors all interacted continuously to vary the manifestations of disease. Just as most men of the cloth failed clearly to demarcate the spheres of God and of material means, so the physician viewed disease as a changed state of being affecting the whole man and capable of being altered by any of his myriad activities.

Even before they had seen cholera, some American physicians wrote soothingly that it was but another form of "sinking typhus," others that it was a variety of bilious fever or a "Lymphatic Hemorrhage." One rural New York doctor cited Benjamin Rush to lend authority to his own classification of cholera as a "suffocated fever."[18]

---

[17] "On the contrary," the author continues, disease "is virtually dis-order, an alteration of the natural state or actions of the tissues or organs of the economy." Hugh L. Hodge, "On the Pathology and Therapeutics of Cholera Maligna," *American Journal of the Medical Sciences*, XII (1833), 388. Hodge cites Broussais and Bichat, and like most American physicians of his day seems not to have assimilated the work of those younger men opposed to Broussais, who sought to define specific clinical entities and whose influence was so great upon the succeeding generation of American physicians.

[18] John Esten Cooke, *op. cit.*, V, 481–500; Thomas Miner, *Boston Medical and Surgical Journal*, VI (August 1, 1832), 397; Diary of William Darrach, August 19, 1832, Pennsylvania Historical Society; E. Cutbush, *Western Medical Gazette*, I (1833), 63.

Most common was the opinion that cholera was only an aggravated form of "cholera morbus"—a flexible term used to describe ailments as diverse as dysentery and diarrhea. Comforting in its familiarity, this nomenclature also played another role, implying a local origin for the disease and, hence, non-importation and non-contagion. In the words of Daniel Drake, cholera bore to "cholera morbus, a relation similar to that of influenza to a common cold." It differed only in virulence. One physician reported finding three or four different degrees of cholera in the same family, ranging from common cholera to the Asiatic or malignant type.[19]

With disease so flexible a concept, it was only natural that mental and moral factors should be presumed to play a role in its causation. Those succumbing to the ubiquitous "epidemic influence" had somehow predisposed themselves, had overeaten, had been intemperate, or had become panic-stricken. Despite the obvious moralism of such injunctions, medical thinkers did not, of course, regard the disease as being a direct imposition of the Lord. Cholera resulted from the physical effect of transgressing natural laws.[20] An active exercise of faith in God and his mercy, for example, would protect one from fear and thus from cholera—but it was "preeminently by the *physical influences* of that faith" that one was protected. For fear has

a more specific operation upon the human body, than any other passion; it spasmodically contracts the mouths of thousands of our perspiring or exhaling vessels, flings the acrid perspirable matter upon the insides of our digestive organs, which it stimulates, and causes by abstracting much of the watery part of our blood, a looseness and congestion in our bowels, the very proximate cause of the Epidemic Cholera.

[19] Daniel Drake, *Western Journal of Medical and Physical Science*, VI (1832), 79; James McNaughton, *Letter on the Epidemic Cholera of Albany* ... (Albany, 1832).

[20] See, for example, Thomas Spencer, "Annual Address, on the Nature of the Epidemic, Usually Called ASIATIC CHOLERA ...," *Transactions of the Medical Society of the State of New York*, 1832–33, p. 220.

Indeed the entire epidemic might be understood as a mass psychological phenomenon akin to the "jerks" at a camp meeting. William Beaumont was only expressing a medical truism of his time, when he wrote that "the Greater proportional number of deaths in the cholera epidemics are, in my opinion, caused more by fright and presentiment of death than from the fatal tendency . . . of the disease."[21]

Despite the attention given to the problems of prophylaxis and treatment, the medical debate which generated the most emotion was that over the possibly contagious nature of cholera. For if cholera were contagious, it would define the conduct of the whole community: how the hospitals were to be organized, what prophylactic measures were to be emphasized, and, most important, whether a quarantine was to be instituted—the last a measure which vitally concerned every man of business.

In 1832, few medical men believed that cholera was a contagious disease. Its cause lay in the atmosphere.[22] The more precise attributed the disease either to some change in the normal constituents of the atmosphere or in the addition to it of some deleterious substance of terrestrial origin.

A greater number found such intellectual refinements un-

[21] The paragraph quoted above, typical of many, is from C. L. Seeger, *A Lecture on the Epidemic Cholera* . . . (Boston, 1832), p. 25; Jesse S. Mayer, *Life and Letters of Dr. William Beaumont* (St. Louis, 1912), pp. 142–43.

[22] A sample of the opinions expressed by 109 American physicians during the years 1832–34 shows that 90 did not consider the disease to be at all contagious, while only 5 considered the disease to be primarily contagious. The other 14 considered it to be primarily non-contagious but admitted that under some circumstances cholera might become communicable (contingent-contagionism). Of the 87 physicians who clearly expressed their opinion as to the actual cause of the disease, 48 considered it to be due to some substance added to the atmosphere or some change in its constituents. Others, expressing only their opinion that the disease was an "epidemic," may also be presumed to have believed in its atmospheric transmission, since an "epidemic" disease was usually defined as one spread through the atmosphere. Ten physicians regarded the disease as being caused by some substance of "terrene" origin in the atmosphere ("miasmatists"). These opinions have been garnered from books, pamphlets, medical journals, newspapers, diaries, letters, and journals. A similar procedure has been followed for the 1849–54 and 1866 epidemics.

necessary, content to intone such phrases as "epidemic influence," "choleraic distemperature," or "uncontrollable atmospheric peculiarity." There were but few to question. The atmospheric theory was too convenient: flexible and amorphous enough to explain the varied phenomenon of the disease, it served also as a weapon against the "antisocial" and "antiquated" doctrine of contagion. The doctrine of predisposing causes played more than a monitory role; it reinforced the weakest link in the atmospheric theory, explaining how some were stricken while others were not, though all breathed the same atmosphere.

Epidemiological thought in the United States had been conditioned by experience with yellow fever, and the black vomit seemed obviously non-contagious. As was the case with yellow fever, so it was with cholera: there could never be found any pattern within the cases that would support a contagionist argument. Cholera, like yellow fever, seemed to start simultaneously in widely separated parts of a city.

These local concentrations of cases, as well as their often sudden and widely scattered outbreak, seemed strong evidence against contagion and for the atmospheric origin of the disease. A Dr. Kane of Plattsburg, for example, appointed by his community to study cholera in Montreal, became convinced that it was not contagious, for it had descended in many parts of the city simultaneously "like a shower of hail." An American physician, observing the disease in Vienna, concluded that its cause must be some alteration in the atmosphere —the only thing that could have affected so many people at the same time. Daniel Drake reached a similar conclusion after observing the disease in Cincinnati.[23] Concentrations of cholera cases in circumscribed slum areas might be charged either to the moral shortcomings of the victims or to the presence of crowded tenements, decaying filth, resident pigs—to any-

[23] *Evangelist* (New York), June 30, 1832; Charles T. Jackson, "Cholera in Vienna," *Medical Magazine*, I (1832–33), 214; *Chronicle* (Cincinnati), October 13, 1832.

thing which might produce miasmata or somehow vitiate the air needed to maintain normal respiration. Only those so weakened would be attacked by the latent poison in the atmosphere.

Experience with vaccination in smallpox, the one undoubtedly new element in etiological thought in the first third of the nineteenth century, served only to reinforce the dominant anticontagionism. Unable to abandon older ideas, medical thinkers failed to generalize from their experience with vaccination and to assume that a similar, though as yet undiscovered, process might be present in other diseases. Any disease not conforming to the rigid and arbitrary "laws" assigned to smallpox could not be contagious.

Nor was it difficult to show by such analogies that cholera was not contagious. Cholera could be contracted more than once, while a contagious disease—defined in terms of smallpox —could not. Even if cholera, like yellow fever, was transmitted from place to place, it did not seem to be passed "from one body to another, or through the medium of those morbid secretions of the human system which preserve and multiply the sources of infection in contagious diseases." Moreover, smallpox was not influenced by atmospheric and climatic changes as were cholera and other "epidemic diseases" (epidemic diseases being, by definition, atmospheric, not contagious). Regardless of external conditions, all exposed to the poison of smallpox would inevitably fall victim unless they had been vaccinated or had recovered from an attack. This was manifestly not the case with cholera.[24]

Contagionism was, morever, decidedly antisocial. To the socially conscious physician, the doctrine of contagion was in itself an "exciting cause" of the disease. The fear, it was argued, caused by a general belief in cholera's contagiousness

[24] [Patrick Macauley], *How Is the Cholera Propagated? . . .* (London, 1831), p. 6; N.Y.C. Board of Health, *Reports of Hospital Physicians . . .* (New York, 1832), p. 140; *Boston Recorder*, June 27, 1832; Joseph M. Smith, *Discourse on the Epidemic Cholera . . .* (New York, 1831), pp. 24–25.

would not only result in many additional cases, but it would completely disrupt the structure of society. Cities would be deserted; commerce would cease; the sick would be left to die alone and without the simplest comforts.

An equally important reason for the almost universal acceptance of the atmospheric theory was the absence of alternatives. The animalcular theory, subject of so much attention by medical historians, was in 1932 merely a variation of standard atmospheric ideas, differing in that the cholera-causing substance in the air was specified as being a "small winged insect not visible to the naked eye." Daniel Drake, the only American physician who held this view in a sample of over a hundred, conceived of the animalcula as "poisonous, invisible, aerial insects, of the same or similar habits with the gnat."[25] This theory, which did recognize the need for assuming some specific material cause for disease and which did suggest that it might be organic, found few converts. It was a notion with "but few enlightened advocates."

Contagionism was the one plausible alternative to the atmospheric theory—and it was in an almost moribund state. In a sample of the opinions of over one hundred American physicians, only one could be found who believed that cholera was invariably contagious.[26] He could be ignored. A sizable minority of physicians, however, believed that in particularly filthy and confined situations the disease might become contagious. These contingent-contagionists, as they were called, had to be shown conclusively that cholera could never be communicated from person to person. Belief in a second cause, they were admonished, when one was sufficient, was "unphilosophical," and reeked of empiricism. (At this time,

[25] Drake, *A Practical Treatise on Epidemic Cholera* (Cincinnati, 1832), p. 44.

[26] Bernard M. Byrne, *An Essay To Prove the Contagious Character of Malignant Cholera* . . . (Baltimore, 1833), pp. 3–4, 7, 9, 59, and *passim*.

significantly, "empiric" was—as it had been for generations—
a synonym for quack.)[27]

American physicians, like most of their European contemporaries, were still thinking in scholastic terms, hoping by
elaborate chains of reasoning to discover the "true philosophy" of a disease. Such reasoning, formal in its rhetoric,
based perhaps on a random observation, recalled the eighteenth century, rather than prefigured the second half of the
nineteenth.

While cholera ravaged Europe in 1831 and the early
months of 1832, American physicians filled newspapers, medical journals, and pamphlets with debate over the necessity of
quarantine. Prevailing medical opinion was decidedly hostile.
The establishment of quarantines would serve merely to "flat-
ter vulgar prejudices," and "embarrass with unnecessary restrictions, the commerce and industry of the country." Energies futilely expended in their enforcement would be diverted from the cleansing and purification that alone could
temper or prevent the disease. Quarantines and sanitary cor-
dons were the engines of oppression, despotism, and bureauc-
racy.[28]

Before the epidemic, however, there was still much opposition to any precipitate discarding of quarantine regulations.

[27] One New Jersey physician, reporting on a group of cholera cases, stated
that though he could not explain them on any basis other than contagion, he
could not consider cholera contagious, for he had seen instances where it
had not spread by contagion, and it was "unphilosophical" to suppose that
there were more causes responsible for a given effect than are absolutely
necessary. S. H. Pennington, "Report for the Eastern District," *Transactions
of the Medical Society of the State of New Jersey*, 1833, p. 308. Dr. Pennington who could not believe the evidence of his own senses is only an extreme
case of a very common view.

[28] C. R. Gilman, *Hints to the People on the Prevention and Early Treat-
ment of Spasmodic Cholera* (New York, 1832), p. 6; Horatio G. Jameson,
"Observations on Epidemic Cholera, as It Appeared at Baltimore, in the
Summer of 1832," *Maryland Medical Recorder*, II (1831), 393; *American
Journal of the Medical Sciences*, X (1832), 204; *Journal of Health*, III
(November 9, 1831), 75–76.

As the editor of the *Boston Medical and Surgical Journal* put
it:

Were the problem of the disease being contagious much less than
it is, it would still be fairly worth considering whether the removal of a probable or even possible source of infection to our
whole population, were not worth a temporary inconvenience to
a few individuals.[29]

By the time cholera had run its course in the United States,
even this moderate position had become indefensible.

The seeming failure of quarantine, and the unpredictable
pattern of cases during the epidemic, brought complete vic-
tory for the anticontagionists. "Non-Contagion," a sardonic
and pseudonymous physician, urged that all those who fur-
thered the "wicked doctrine of contagion, should forthwith
be put *hors de combat*, or delivered over to the keeper of a
cholera or insane asylum." Another cynical medical man declared that existing quarantines were the result of a yielding
by the thinking part of the community to the irrational fears
of the panic-stricken multitude. "Some future historian," he
reflected, "will record our folly and credulity in the same
chapter of events with Salem witchcraft, divining rods, and
animal magnetism."[30]

29 *Boston Medical and Surgical Journal*, V (September 6, 1832), 65.

30 *Evening Post* (New York), July 12, 1832; Christopher C. Yates, *Observations on the Epidemic Now Prevailing in the City of New-York* ... (New
York, 1832), p. 34; Alexander H. Stephens, in a letter to John Collins Warren (July 18, 1832, Warren Papers, Massachusetts Historical Society), characterized the quarantine which he was supposed to help enforce as president
of New York's Special Medical Council as a "useless embarrassment to commerce."
It seems at first thought paradoxical that the idea of contagionism should
have but a few decades before the discoveries of Pasteur and Koch been held
in such low esteem. In an article discussed widely by historians of medicine,
Erwin H. Ackerknecht has attempted to define some of the causal factors in
this apparently anomalous circumstance. As the nineteenth century opened,
he suggests, contagionism seemed a medieval belief, one which had never
been subjected to scientific scrutiny: "It is no accident that so many leading
anti-contagionists were leading scientists. To them this was a fight for science,
against outdated authorities and medieval mysticism; for observation and
research against systems and speculation." Quarantines, the logical result of

The conviction that cholera was not contagious was, however, limited to the medical profession and to the more enlightened among the laity. Most ordinary folk believed that the disease was spread by some specific contagion. Despite the soothing words of physicians, it was almost impossible to rent even the meanest sort of building for use as a cholera hospital. It was equally difficult to hire nurses to work in them.

Some intelligent and articulate lay observers, not burdened with the theoretical knowledge of the medical men, were also impressed with evidences of contagion. Charles Francis Adams noted in his diary that the disease followed the tracks of commerce, which "would seem to sustain the doctrine of contagion." To shrewd old Deborah Logan, chronicler of Philadelphia society, contagion was too apparent to be doubted. To respectable New Yorkers like John Pintard and Philip Hone, it seemed quite likely that the disease was communicable.[31] Not to have enforced quarantines would have been politically suicidal.

---

a belief in contagion "meant to the rapidly growing classes of merchants and industrialists, a source of losses, a limitation to expansion, a weapon of bureaucratic control that it was no longer willing to tolerate. Contagionism would, through its association with the old bureaucratic powers, be suspect to all liberals, trying to reduce state interference to a minimum." ("Anti-Contagionism between 1821 and 1867," *Bulletin of the History of Medicine*, XXII [1948], 567.) In America, it might be added, the omnipresent rhetoric of progress and democracy neatly allied itself with a tender concern for the needs of commerce. Indeed, there could be no conflict, for trade was progress, and there could be no progress without trade.

[31] Diary of Charles Francis Adams, June 24, 1832, microfilm, Columbia University Library; Diary of Deborah Norris Logan, August 4, 1832, Manuscript Division, Pennsylvania Historical Society; Pintard, *Letters from John Pintard to His Daughter Eliza Noel Pintard Davidson, 1816–1833* (New York, 1941), IV, 78; Diary of Philip Hone, September 20, 1832, Manuscript Division, New York Historical Society.

V. ALDERMEN AND CHOLERA

Cholera could not be ignored. Medicines, nursing, and hospitals must be provided for the sick. The dead must be buried, the orphans cared for. Houses, streets, and lots must be inspected, cleaned, and disinfected, and the common people guarded against themselves, made to understand that it would mean death to continue their ordinary habits in cholera times. All this demanded money, money and organization, and the co-operation of government, physicians, and citizens.

Until relatively recent times, leadership during epidemics has come almost invariably from outside established administrative circles. Temporary committees, organized and led by the more courageous members of the community, exercised the functions of a paralyzed municipal government. As soon as the epidemic declined in virulence, these committees began spontaneously to disintegrate, leaving behind no permanent organization to prevent or cope with future outbreaks. This traditional pattern continued unbroken until well into the nineteenth century; America's most famous epidemic—Philadelphia's encounter with yellow fever in 1793—exhibited perfectly the workings of such a surrogate government. For two months, a city almost in chaos was administered by a completely unofficial group of public-spirited citizens.[1]

[1] For an excellent account of this epidemic, see John H. Powell, *Bring Out Your Dead: The Great Plague of Yellow Fever in Philadelphia in 1793* (Philadelphia, 1949).

State and municipal governments had grown in experience and power in the forty years between 1793 and 1832. A dozen bouts with yellow fever during these same years had prepared and conditioned New York City for its struggle with cholera. During the summer of 1832, its Board of Health was able to assume, at least temporarily, many of the functions of the twentieth-century government—hospital and welfare services, slum clearance, and food and drug control. Informal responses to overwhelming necessity, however, these functions were as short-lived as the epidemic which created them.

The Board of Health was quite conscious of the role it should have to fill were cholera to appear in New York City and had begun to take what preventive measures it could almost a year before the disease crossed the Atlantic. The board organized a committee to gather information, urged the national government to send a medical commission to Europe, and enforced quarantine throughout the winter of 1831–32.[2]

The day after the news that cholera had broken out in Canada became known (June 16), the board met to formulate a program to protect the city. They resolved that the city councilmen should act as health wardens for their own wards, with full power to enforce the directives of the board, and agreed to send a commission to Montreal and Quebec. Before adjourning, the board also appointed a committee to inquire into the nature and extent of its powers.[3]

A few days later, this committee reported encouragingly that the powers of the board were, under existing statutes, "full and ample to meet every emergency." In the presence of "epidemic or pestilential disease," it had the power to regulate

---

[2] See chap. i.

[3] New York City Board of Health, Minutes, June 16, 1832, Municipal Archives and Records Center (hereinafter cited as Minutes). It will be recalled that the Board of Health consisted of the Board of Aldermen meeting with the mayor and recorder.

internal as well as external commerce, impose a quarantine on individuals, and "exercise all such other powers . . . as in their judgment the circumstances of the case and the public good shall require." It was the board, moreover, which decided when a disease was "epidemic or pestilential," and thus when these broad powers could be exercised.[4] The report concluded by warning that all actions of the board should be made by its official agents. Its two regular employees were, of course, unable to perform the countless tasks demanded by the epidemic. To meet day-to-day needs, the board depended upon administrative expedients, temporary personnel, and the co-operation of the permanent agencies of the municipality, such as the Commissioners of the Alms-House and the standing committees of the City Council.

The most important of the board's administrative expedients was the Special Medical Council, created early in July by the Board of Health and manned by seven of the city's more prominent physicians. Since the board was, with one accidental exception, composed of laymen, it was the Special Medical Council that made the key decisions in fighting the epidemic, decisions enforced by committees of the Board of Health.

These committees, usually consisting of three members, implemented all of the board's decisions. When, for example, it was decided to rent several buildings to house the poor removed from their slum homes, a three-man committee was formed. These three aldermen, "with power," spent several days inspecting dozens of buildings and haggling with as many landlords before making final arrangements and reporting their results. The board had a kind of amoeba-like existence, extruding temporary "organs" as it required them.

The most important of these was a three-man committee to which the executive powers of the board had been dele-

[4] Report of the Committee Appointed To Report on the Powers of the Board, City Clerk's Papers, File Drawer U-57, Municipal Archives and Records Center.

gated.[5] This special Executive Committee supervised the purchase and distribution of supplies to the hospitals and dispensaries, the hiring and firing of doctors and nurses, and scores of other minor, but necessary, tasks. More frequently than not, it was the Executive Committee that put into effect the decisions of the Special Medical Council. When their medical advisors urged the board to forbid the sale of fruit or submitted their nominations for hospital physicians, these communications were referred to the Executive Committee.

The ward was the practical basis of administration. Physicians and dispensaries were assigned by ward, as were all appropriations for relief and sanitation. Only the hospitals were established without reference to ward divisions. In each of the city's fifteen wards, the alderman and assistant alderman, acting as health wardens, organized and supervised the purification of streets and houses and in many cases provided for the care of the sick. However, the advantages of personal familiarity and responsibility which this system provided were offset by equally obvious disadvantages. The councilmen were elected officials before they were health wardens, and could ill-afford to ignore the demands of practical politics. Nepotism and political considerations influenced medical appointments.[6] The board could never bring itself to take any action against the saloons—and their political co-workers, the saloonkeepers—although medical opinion was unanimous in denouncing their continued existence. Appropriations had to be the same for every ward, although their needs differed widely.

[5] This committee was originally created (Minutes, July 3, 1832) to provide accommodations for the sick "in the public hospitals or elsewhere." The Minutes for February 18, 1833, show that the Executive Committee spent $67,544.63 of the city's total expenditure of $117,687.41 in fighting the epidemic.

[6] James R. Manley, for instance, later claimed that the appointment of the Special Medical Council was merely part of a plot by the recorder, Richard Riker, to oust him from his position as resident physician, so that his (Riker's) son-in-law could be appointed instead. James R. Manley, *Letters Addressed to the Board of Health . . .* (New York, 1832).

Fortunately, city finances were adequate to the emergency. The funds used by the Board of Health to combat the epidemic came from the city treasury, and no special appeals or loans were needed.[7] In theory, funds had to be appropriated by the Common Council and then allotted by the comptroller to the Board of Health. Actually, during the summer of 1832, the board was spending money much faster than it was being appropriated. (The Board of Assistant Aldermen was not, as yet, a part of the Board of Health, and their assent was required for appropriations.) There was an undoubted helter-skelter in its finances. Myndert Van Schaick, the treasurer, had to spend several hundred dollars of his own to settle accounts; and dozens of lawsuits remained to be settled after the epidemic.[8]

Months before the city had had to care for its first case of cholera, thinking New Yorkers were conscious of the need for providing hospitals, medicine, and doctors for the city's poor. Nevertheless, it was not until the evening of July 4 that the Board of Health's first makeshift cholera hospital opened its doors.[9] The board had had to start from scratch in providing for the sick. The operation of hospitals, as distinct from almshouses, was not, at this time, considered a municipal responsibility; and the trustees of New York's one private

---

[7] Minutes, February 18, 1833, contain a summary of the municipal disbursements:

To the several wards	$ 41,144.73
To the several almshouses	6,546.28
To the hospitals	45,173.08
To the Special Medical Council	7,748.00
To miscellaneous objects	16,096.23
To chloride of lime—on hand	979.09
Total	$117,687.41

[8] N.Y.C. Board of Assistants, *Report of the Special Committee, to Whom Was Referred the Two Resolutions of Alderman Van Schaick . . .* , Doc. No. 49 (New York, 1832).

[9] N.Y.C. Board of Health, *Reports of Hospital Physicians . . .* (New York, 1832), pp. 11–12. By September, the five hospitals that the city had eventually established had treated 2,030 patients. An additional 555 cases were treated at the Bellevue Almshouse.

hospital had refused to accept cholera patients. Despite the earnest solicitations of the board, James DePeyster, Philip Hone, and the other governors of New York Hospital decided that their bylaws forbade the hospital to patients suffering from "infectious diseases."[10]

The temporary hospitals of the board were a makeshift and ill-assorted set of buildings: a school, a bank, the half-completed Hall of Records. The hospital at Corlear's Hook was an old workshop which

when first opened for the reception of patients . . . was without a sash or pane of glass to the windows, and the weather boards and doors were full of cracks and crevices, through which winds and rain were freely admitted. It required several days before it could be made tight, clean, and comfortable, as two carpenters only could be induced to work among the sick and dying. For the first few days after opening the hospital there was much irregularity, noises and confusion from men engaged in whitewashing the interior of the building; from carpenters at work inside and out; and from the press of patients, received, dying, and in agonies with cramps and vomiting.[11]

Few, understandably, wished to live near one of these hospitals. Workers in a shipyard adjoining the Corlear's Hook Hospital left work so unanimously and precipitately at its establishment that their employers were unable to fulfil their contracts. The opinion of these humble shipwrights was shared by most of their betters.[12]

Preventing the disease was even more important than caring for those unfortunates who had already fallen victim: the acknowledged first duty of the government in protecting the

[10] Diary of Philip Hone, July 5, 1832, Manuscript Division, New York Historical Society; Minutes, July 5, 8, 1832.

[11] N.Y.C. Board of Health, *Reports of Hospital Physicians* . . . , p. 112.

[12] Cf. Trustees of the Public Schools to Mayor Bowne, n.d., Filed Papers of the Common Council, File Drawer T-594, Municipal Archives and Records Center; *Truth Teller* (New York), August 11, 1832; Minutes, August 25, September 12, 1832; John W. Casilear to John Kensett, July 8, 1832, Edwin D. Morgan Papers, Manuscript Division, New York State Library.

public health was to cleanse and "purify" streets and houses.
New York's Board of Health spent a good proportion of its
time during the summer of 1832 in seeing that the streets,
lots, cellars, and docks were denuded of their decades' accumulation of filth. With some exceptions, the streets were
cleaner and less noisome than they had been at any time within the memory of New Yorkers.

How surprised, then, were the citizens of New York . . . to behold the tidiness of their streets. "Where in the world did all these
stones come from?" said one old lady who had lived all her life in
the city; "I never knew that the streets were covered with stones
before. How very droll!"[13]

But this cleanliness, so marked in some sections of the city,
was not to be found at all in others. At the height of the
epidemic, a house at 31 Renwick Street was found to have in
its yard "from forty to fifty hogs, four cows, and two horses,"
and to be "so filthy that the first physician called . . . refused
to enter."[14]

The Board of Health and its medical advisors, following
precedents formed during a generation of yellow fever epidemics, felt that the lives of the poor could be saved only by
depopulating the city's worst slums; and they *were* evacuated,
despite the lawsuits of anguished landlords. With Bellevue a
pesthouse, the Board of Health was faced with the necessity
of finding housing for the indigent and now homeless poor.
In characteristic fashion, it created a Committee to Provide
Suitable Accommodations for the Destitute Poor. Within a
few days of their appointment, its three members could report
to the board (July 14) that they had rented several buildings,
hired attendants, and arranged with the Executive Committee
and the Commissioners of the Alms-House for the supply of
food, medicines, and clothing. In addition to the two brick
buildings that they had rented, the committee had had "ranges
of shanties" erected in a half-dozen places in the city.

13 [Asa Greene], *A Glance at New York* . . . (New York, 1837), pp. 173,
175.
14 *Commercial Advertiser* (New York), July 25, 1832.

This housing seems to have been something less than satisfactory. Hastily thrown-together shanties were ill-suited to
the preservation of health; those at Tenth Street and Avenue
C, "for the accommodation of colored people in health," were
so leaky that the first rainstorm completely soaked the inhabitants and their belongings.[15] Rents paid for several buildings
were extortionate; and the budget-conscious Executive Committee, speaking for many New Yorkers, was quick to criti-
cize arrangements that provided the poor with food, clothing,
and lodgings and yet allowed them to "wander about the city
all day in great measure indifferent whether they find employ
or not." All further aid, they concluded, should be given
through the Commissioners of the Alms-House.[16]

However, the Commissioners of the Alms-House—proto-
type of the modern welfare department—were already over-
burdened. Their resources were inadequate to the task of providing subsistence for the families of thousands of wage earn-
ers thrown out of work by the abrupt cessation of the city's
business. Though the commissioners had erected temporary
buildings on their grounds and were issuing rations to some
of the unemployed, at least half of the relief work was being
undertaken by private citizens, churches, and the well-organized Committee of the Benevolent. This latter group, divided
into fifteen subcommittees corresponding to the city's fifteen
wards, had embarked upon a comprehensive program of aid.
They paid the poor for sewing and "for cleansing and purify-
ing their own dwellings." The committee established soup
kitchens in each ward. In the Fifth Ward, for example, the
poor could get meat, soup, and bread from ten to four o'clock
on the North Battery at the foot of Hubert Street.[17]

There were those who felt that such activities were the
concern of the municipal government, "the legitimate father

[15] *Evening Post* (New York), July 27, 1832; Minutes, July 14, 1832.

[16] Executive Committee to the Board of Health, August 10, 1832, City
Clerk's Papers, File Drawer U-59, Municipal Archives and Records Center.

[17] The daily newspapers carried the notices of the several ward committees, telling where foods and medicines might be obtained.

of the poor of this city."[18] But it was their criticism, and not the procedure, which was new. This mixture of public and private charity was accepted in times of crisis—in the embargo period, for example, or during the yellow fever epidemics of 1798, 1805, and 1822.

A constant source of embarrassment to the Board of Health was the admitted inaccuracy of the cholera reports that they issued. Official statements continued to be unreliable even after doctors had been threatened with a fifty-dollar fine for each unreported case of cholera.[19] More dangerous were the disgraceful conditions at the Potter's Field and at St. Patrick's cemetery. Dead bodies lay unburied for days before being thrown into shallow pits and covered with a foot or two of loose earth, which served neither to keep the rats out nor the odors of putrefaction in. In response to dozens of complaints, the Board of Health directed the keeper of the Potter's Field to bury the dead no more than three deep and to cover the top tier of coffins with at least six inches of quicklime and five feet of earth. Conditions at St. Patrick's were at least as bad. The entrance to the vault was found to have been *"partially closed by an old door* surrounded by thousands of flies, and the *stench from it unbearable."*[20]

Day after day, throughout the summer of 1832, the Board of Health absorbed the almost unanimous criticism of indignant New Yorkers. And much of it was justified. While some of the city's streets were so clean as to be unrecognizable, others seem never to have been touched by a broom. On this score, the board can be defended, for the practical difficulties

18 *Cholera Bulletin,* July 20, 1832. This passage is also cited in David Schneider, *The History of Public Welfare in New York State, 1609–1866* (Chicago, 1938), p. 256.

19 The same penalty was imposed for the same offense in previous yellow fever epidemics. Cf. James Hardie, *An Account of the Malignant Fever Which Prevailed in the City of New York, during the Autumn of 1805* (New York, 1805), p. 32.

20 Minutes, July 22, 29, 1832; Henry Wyckoff to the Board of Health, July 7, 1832, City Clerk's Papers, File Drawer U-58, Municipal Archives and Records Center.

of undoing the neglect of decades was enormous. There can be no real defense for the lack of courage and foresight that the board members displayed in refusing to acknowledge the presence of the disease or in their waiting until cholera was already upon them to set up hospitals. Despite bold words affirming the adequacy of their powers, the board lacked the precedents, the imagination, and the disinterest to use them fully.

Americans were unrivaled joiners. Every misstep by the Board of Health provoked a flurry of letters suggesting that its functions be assumed by "combinations of citizens." Still, the struggle of New York against cholera was carried out almost entirely by the regularly constituted municipal authorities. The same was true of Boston, Philadelphia, Baltimore—of almost every one of America's cities.

This seeming commonplace is not without significance. American cities were no longer hypertrophied villages, and their governments had begun to assume the powers necessary for dealing with the problems which their growth had made inevitable. Outside of the largest cities, however, municipal governments were in a far more rudimentary state and were ill-equipped to cope unaided with a threat so disruptive as cholera.

The problem of finance was almost insurmountable for many small towns and even good-sized cities. A community as small as Albany spent over $19,000 in public funds in fighting the epidemic. What city besides Boston could, or would, appropriate $50,000 at the mere whisper of cholera? Raising the money to pay physicians, to hire health wardens and street-cleaners, and to purchase medicines and chloride of lime represented a financial crisis to even flourishing communities. In Newark, New Jersey, and Kingston, New York, citizens at public meetings promised to make good any money spent by their health boards. In many New England towns, meetings were called to authorize expenditures. Cincinnati could scrape up no funds at all for cleansing; and in desperation, Cincinnatians proposed that several dozen of the largest taxpayers come forward, pay their taxes early, and thus provide funds for the Board of Health. The St. Louis treasury was so empty that it would have been impossible to clean the city without the authorization of a special loan. Most small towns and villages avoided the problem by spending almost no money, the health officer and health wardens volunteering their services.[21]

Few towns, however large, had regular boards of health. A city as progressive as Boston created a special Board of Health Commissioners late in June, 1832, but its life was limited to six months.[22] In New York, it will be recalled, the state legislature was forced to pass a special act enabling towns and incorporated villages to form such bodies. In some cities, like Nashville, Tennessee, the Board of Health was identical with the local medical society. More frequently, the board consisted of several members of the city government meeting with the physicians of the town. In many other communities, as in New York, the mayor and other elected officials acted as a board of health. Smaller towns often chose volunteer health committees at public meetings.

Almost everywhere, private citizens formed impromptu organizations to aid public authorities in efforts to combat the epidemic. In New England, town meetings authorized the expenditures and approved the policies of their local health boards. In other towns, public meetings endorsed or attacked board of health policies, and formed voluntary committees to help fight the epidemic. Cities were divided into districts, wards into subwards, their residents volunteering to search them thoroughly for nuisances, to care for the sick, and to collect and distribute food, clothing, and money for the poor.

21 Albany Finance Department, *Report of the Chamberlain . . . of the Expenses Incurred by the Board of Health, of the City of Albany during the Prevalence of the Cholera* (Albany, 1832), p. 3; *Independent Chronicle* (Boston), August 1, 1832; *Monitor* (Newark), July 3, 1832; *Sentinel of Freedom* (Newark), June 26, 1832; *Ulster Palladium* (Kingston, N.Y.), June 20, 1832; *Chronicle* (Cincinnati), September 22, 1832; and *Beacon* (St. Louis), September 20, 1832.

22 Boston City Council, *Ordered . . . June 20, 1832* (Boston, 1832), p. 3.

Boston, thorough, virtuous, and public-spirited as usual, boasted what was probably the most elaborate such organization. The Boston Relief Association consisted of thirteen ward committees directed by a central committee. Members could be transferred from one ward to another, though they could not absent themselves without an excuse. Aid was to be rendered to the sick, but in a manner that should "avoid even the appearance of ostentation or officiousness." In other cities, Rochester and Washington, for example, boards of health appointed ward committees to collect and distribute aid for the poor. Broadsides proclaimed that ladies might be requested as well to form committees to care for widows and orphans.[23]

The true philanthropist had other responsibilities. Perhaps most important was his obligation not to flee and throw those dependent upon him out of work. "Is it *morally right* thus to inflict utter misery and ruin upon others, for a contingent benefit to ourselves?"[24] Nor did the responsibility end with the mere providing of work. Those having charge of laboring men were urged to "institute the most wholesome regulations as to regimen and diet, and act as fathers of families, and there will be much less danger from hard and continued labor than from relaxation, indolence, idleness and indulgence."[25] Dwellers in communities unscathed by the epidemic could show their concern by contributing to the poor in stricken areas.

The same problems faced each community, whether it had an elaborate board of health or merely a makeshift committee of citizens. First, attempts must be made to prevent the disease. Here, despite the scorn of the medically enlightened, the most important step was that of instituting a quarantine. Coastal cities, lake ports, and canal and river towns of whatever size enforced quarantines. Rhode Island proclaimed

[23] Boston Relief Association, *Regulations of the Boston Relief Association, with a List of Members* (Boston, 1832), p. 5–7; *Republican* (Rochester), August 14, 1832; City of Washington, "Cholera," September 5, 1832, Broadsides, Portfolio 194, No. 32, Library of Congress.

[24] *Banner of the Church* (Boston), August 25, 1832.

[25] *Christian Intelligencer* (New York), June 23, 1832.

"martial law," with the governor having wide powers including that of taking "requisite" money from the treasury. The administration of such quarantine must have been a severe strain to many small communities. Troy, for instance, an Erie Canal town, was forced to provide for some seven hundred quarantined immigrants.[26]

The towns themselves had to be cleaned. And it was no easy task to remove tons of encrusted dirt with carts, shovels, and brooms. Even if this conglomerate of rotting garbage, dead animals, and excrement was removed from streets and lots, what could be done with it? In New York, it was thrown into the river. In many inland towns, it was merely taken a few hundred yards outside the corporate limits and there deposited to rot in the sun and fill the atmosphere with the noxious miasmas which, it was believed, lowered men's vitality and predisposed them to disease. Only Boston seemed to have been conspicuously successful in its ablutions.[27] In most places, the clean-up ended with the municipal filth undisturbed, but covered with a reassuring layer of chloride of lime.

Hospitals, nurses, and physicians had to be provided for the poor. And this was no simple task; the establishments fitted up for cholera patients provoked widespread distaste. Neighbors resorted to everything from humble petitions to arson in their efforts to have them removed. Not that respectable folk opposed cholera hospitals. Everyone agreed they were necessary—but on someone else's street.

A cholera hospital, like an almshouse, was an institution for those who could afford no better; death in a cholera hospital was evidence of a life misspent. "The visitor," it was reported, "finds few others in those receptables than the impenetrable

26 *Ohio State Journal* (Columbus), June 30, 1832, prints the proclamation of Governor Duncan MacArthur dated June 28; C. S. J. Goodrich, "Cholera at Troy, New York," *Cholera Gazette*, I (September 19, 1832), 166 ff.

27 John Collins Warren recalled that the city had never had such a thorough cleaning, and never again returned to the filthy condition in which it had been before 1832. Edward Warren, *The Life of John Collins Warren, M.D. . . .* (Boston, 1860), I, 256. Other accounts, however, suggest that the city was not long in returning to its accustomed condition.

sot and debauchee." It was, protested one physician, unfair
that the "respectable" poor should have to be treated in cholera hospitals and not in their homes. Prospective patients were
terrified of them. One old woman in New York's Five Points
preferred, she said, to die locked in her miserable apartment
than to be taken away to perish in unfamiliar surroundings
and at the hands of callous strangers. The poor were quite
certain as well that once in these "slaughterhouses," they
would become the helpless subjects for the experiments of
eager young physicians. In Utica, an infuriated mob of Irish
workingmen stormed the cholera hospital; and even in enlightened Philadelphia, physicians and attendants were vilified
and abused.[28]

Nurses were almost impossible to find. It was dirty work,
and despite the reassurances of physicians, dangerous. (At
New York's Greenwich Hospital, fourteen of sixteen nurses
died of cholera contracted while caring for patients.) Offers
of exorbitant salaries attracted only "mercenaries, who appear to possess as little sympathy or humanity as the walls."
In Philadelphia's Arch Street Prison, the inmates cared for
each other. The same was true at many almshouses where no
money could be spared for nurses. In Lexington, Kentucky,
nurses could not be obtained at any salary, with the result
that no cholera hospital was established. Hagerstown, Maryland, avoided this problem by establishing a hospital without
attendants. Visitors to hospitals were often pressed into service and the benevolent urged to volunteer their labor. Only
the Sisters of Charity could be depended upon to serve faithfully; in Philadelphia, Baltimore, Louisville, St. Louis, and
Cincinnati, they staffed the cholera hospitals, working with
little sleep or food until the epidemic subsided.[29]

[28] *Christian Mirror* (Portland, Me.), August 2, 1832; John Thomson, *A
Philosophical Theory of an "Empiric," Proved Practically* . . . (Albany,
1833), p. 5; *Utica Observer*, n.d., cited in *National Intelligencer* (Washington, D.C.), September 11, 1832; Board of Medical Advisers to the Philadelphia Sanitary Committee, August 6, 1832, *Saturday Courier* (Philadelphia),
August 11, 1832.

[29] Alexander H. Stevens, "On the Communicability of Asiatic Cholera,"

With personal habits conceded to be a major cause of cholera, it was the duty of a public health board to protect the
poor and vicious from themselves. It was necessary, as a Connecticut physician demanded, that boards of health have "the
power to *change the habits of the sensual, the vicious, the
intemperate.*"[30] And in America in 1832, there were many
willing to undertake so godly a task.

In the four decades before the Civil War, America was a
holy land upon whose soil were waged the battles of number-
less crusaders for the millennium. Sin in all of its manifestations, from slavery to corsets, was enfiladed by a generation
of self-assured moral reformers. To these zealots, cholera
seemed but a dramatic testament to the pertinence of their
particular cause. Strict Sabbatarians felt that the prevalence
of the disease was "owing to vices which a proper regard to
the Sabbath would check more effectually than anything
else."[31] Health reformers like the Grahamites and social reformers of all sorts managed to find convenient object lessons
in the prevailing epidemic, but none with the success of the
vociferous and well-organized temperance advocates.

Whiskey, temperance orators charged, was directly responsible for one-half of all madness, one-half of all sudden death,
and one-fourth of all adult deaths. Drink itself could cause
almost any disease from cancer to rheumatism, while the
drunkard himself, as Charles Caldwell put it, was "as truly a
monomaniac, as he who, sound in his other conceptions, be-

Transactions of the Medical Society of the State of New York, 1850, p. 36;
"A," *Liberal Advocate* (Rochester), August 4, 1832; Pennsylvania House of
Representatives, *Report of the Committee Appointed To Investigate the
Local Causes of Cholera in the Arch Street Prison . . .* (Harrisburg, 1833),
p. 200; Lunsford P. Yandell, *Transylvania Journal of Medicine*, VI, 200;
Free Press (Hagerstown), n.d., cited in the *Enquirer* (Richmond), October
2, 1832.

[30] Amariah Brigham, *A Treatise on Epidemic Cholera* (Hartford, 1832),
p. 338.

[31] *Mercury* (New York), July 25, 1832.

lieves his feet and legs to be made of glass or butter, or his head of copper."[32]

The doctrine of predisposing causes lent scientific plausibility to the claims of the temperance reformers; it seemed obvious that, with a cholera influence in the atmosphere, the saloons were literally being allowed to dispense poison. A number of communities finally did forbid the sale of intoxicating beverages for the duration of the epidemic.[33] General Scott, commanding American troops in their expedition against Black Hawk, ordered that any soldier found intoxicated should, as soon as he was sober, be forced to dig his own grave.[34]

At least one physician felt in retrospect that the cholera epidemic had been fortunate, for it had made unmistakable the connection between strong drink and disease. A New Jersey practitioner, noting that the drunkards within his purview seemed, if anything, more immune than the temperate, resolved not to circulate his perverse observation. "If it not be so in fact, still, for the sake of temperance and good order, let it stand that the drunkard is peculiarly the victim of cholera."[35] Physicians prepared to question the connection between cholera and drink knew that they would gain only criticism for their scientific scruples. Moral imperatives were still foremost in the American mind.

Almost as dangerous as alcohol were coarse and indigestible

[32] Caldwell, "Thoughts on the Pathology, Prevention and Treatment of Intemperance, as a Form of Mental Derangement," *Transylvania Medical Journal*, V (1832), 330.

[33] Washington, D.C., Cleveland, and Haverhill, Massachusetts, were three communities which did so. Cf. *Liberator* (Boston), August 18, 1832; *Western Luminary* (Lexington, Ky.), July 25, 1832; John A. Krout, *The Origins of Prohibition* (New York, 1925), pp. 232–33.

[34] Frank E. Stevens, *The Blackhawk War* (Chicago, 1903), pp. 248–49.

[35] S. H. Pennington, *Transactions of the Medical Society of New Jersey*, 1833, p. 308. R. Nelson, in *Asiatic Cholera* (New York, 1866), p. 64, recalled that as health commissioner of Montreal in 1832, he was warned against announcing that cholera did not seem to be any more prevalent among drunkards. Daniel Drake experienced similar pressures in Cincinnati.

foods. It was easier to offend the market gardeners, fish-mongers, and butchers than the saloonkeepers, and in almost every community in which cholera prevailed, the sale of at least some foods was forbidden. In New York, for example, the Market Committee banned the sale of "green and unripe fruits of every kind, and more especially of gooseberries, ap-ples, pears, and also of cucumbers and green corn." Despite the jibes of the facetious, most Americans believed implicitly that a green apple or a roasting ear, when eaten in a "cholera at-mosphere" was equivalent to that much arsenic. In Baltimore, it was reported that a laboring man upon returing home found his wife and children about to eat a watermelon. He warned them against eating it and gave the melon to a hog, which died promptly of cholera.[36] Only the poor, who could not afford to vary their diet, returned each day with their market baskets filled with the forbidden—though plentiful—fruit.

It would be comforting to close this chapter on an optimis-tic note, to dwell on a series of public-spirited and enlightened reforms resulting from the epidemic. Unfortunately, this is impossible. Boards of health evaporated as abruptly as they had come into being. The modest measures of cleanliness which New York had attained in the summer of 1832 did not outlast the heat of August as the Board of Health settled into its customary apathy.[37] For a few years—and especially dur-ing the minor cholera epidemic of 1834—it met more regu-larly and attempted to institute some of the public health measures which the city needed so badly. But the board never did institute such reforms and, by 1836, was functioning pre-cisely as it had in 1831, meeting irregularly and existing in a kind of administrative latency. It awaited the stimulus of a new epidemic to bring it to life.

---

[36] *Evening Post* (New York), July 30, 1832; *Palladium* (New Haven), September 13, 1832. This, of course, was the sort of story ridiculed by the more irreverent. Cf. *Sentinel* (New York), August 27, 28, 1832; *Constellation* (New York), Sept. 1, 1832.

[37] See *American for the Country* (New York), September 4, 1832.

PART 2

1849

VI. THE EPIDEMIC: 1849

Twenty-two days out of Havre, the packet ship "New York" dropped anchor at quarantine late Friday night, December 1, 1848. Early the next morning, New York's deputy health officer rowed out to inspect the new arrival and her 331 steerage passengers.

An alarmed captain greeted him with the report that seven immigrants had died below decks. Others were sick, exhibiting the unmistakable symptoms of cholera. It was no routine report which his deputy presented to Dr. John Sterling, the health officer.[1] But it could have come as no great surprise.

Cholera, like revolution, had swept through Europe in 1848. Spreading outward from its Ganges homeland, the disease had, in a half-dozen years, visited almost every part of Asia, Europe, and the Middle East. In July, 1847, it was in Astrakhan, a year later in Berlin; early in October of 1848 it appeared in London. In the fall of 1848, as in the spring of 1832, cholera poised at the Atlantic.

Realistic Americans assumed that this barrier would not long protect the United States. The course of the epidemic was the same as it had been in 1832, except that the Atlantic

[1] John W. Sterling, "History of the Asiatic Cholera at Quarantine, Staten Island, New-York, in December, 1848, and January, 1849," *New York Journal of Medicine*, III (1849), 9.

was now crossed more rapidly, more frequently, and by larger ships. With cholera in London and Edinburgh in October, diarist George Templeton Strong commented resignedly, it would doubtless be in New York before the New Year.[2]

By mid-October, the medically sophisticated had already begun to notice forerunners of cholera in the atmosphere. Insects swarmed, influenza and diarrheas were epidemic, and the usual diseases of winter failed to respond to treatment.[3] In this tainted air, the decades' accumulation of filth that polluted houses, streets, and yards was more than ordinarily pernicious. To allow the continued existence of such breeding places of pestilence seemed inexcusable, and moribund health boards and street-cleaning committees were attacked for their chronic inactivity. In Philadelphia the Board of Health, in Boston the City Council, and in Baltimore the Medical and Chirurgical Society had, by December, begun to prepare for the epidemic.[4] Again, as in 1832, the reports of medical commissions filled hundreds of columns in newspapers and medical journals.

Though disquieting in their methodical description of agony and death, these reports provided some reassurance. They bore repeated testimony to the relative immunity of the well-nourished, the prudent, and the temperate. Nor, the reports agreed, did the disease seem as severe in this its second tour of Europe. New Englanders were especially soothed by a plausible new theory which held that cholera flourished only in areas underlain by limestone. Perhaps this explained

2 *The Diary of George Templeton Strong* (New York, 1952), I, 332.

3 *Boston Investigator*, October 11, 1848; *Niles' National Register*, LXXIV (September 6, 1848), 145; William M. McPheeters, "History of the Epidemic Cholera in St. Louis in 1849," *St. Louis Medical and Surgical Journal*, VII (1850), 97–98.

4 As early as September, the Philadelphia Board of Health had communicated with the Boston City Council in regard to the impending epidemic. Boston Board of Health, *Report of the Committee of Internal Health on the Asiatic Cholera . . .* , City Document No. 66 (Boston, 1849), p. 4; Eugene F. Cordell, *The Medical Annals of Maryland, 1799–1899* (Baltimore, 1903), p. 120.

how granite-bound New England escaped so lightly in 1832. Most reassuring of all was the unshaken conviction that the United States was the most prosperous, pious, and enlightened of nations. Cholera's ancestral home was India, its natural victims a dirty, ignorant, and fatalistic people.[5]

There was little doubt in the minds of medical men, however, that cholera could thrive wherever there was sufficient filth. And no extraordinary sensibilities were required to see and smell the potential death in America's cities and villages. Few communities could provide their citizens with a reliable supply of water;[6] sanitation and waste disposal were everywhere inadequate. Pigs, dogs, and goats still provided the only effective sanitation in many American cities. Pigs in the streets, like Brother Jonathan and the Indians, were an ineradicable part of the European image of the United States.

The hogs roamed everywhere. In New York pig-naping became a recognized trade (practiced by men who toured the city in wagons, scooping up unwatched pigs and selling them to butchers). In Little Rock, Arkansas, the porkers filled the streets and had, as one editor put it, begun to "dispute the side walks with *other persons*." Such whimsey could not be shared by the parents of children killed or mutilated by foraging pigs.[7]

[5] For an exposition of the "limestone theory," see the *Journal* (Boston), November 24, 1848. For the idea that the epidemic was less severe than its counterpart in 1832, see *Connecticut Courant* (Hartford), December 2, 1848; *Olive Branch* (Boston), January 6, 1849; *Public Ledger* (Philadelphia), December 8, 1848; *American* (Rochester), December 5, 1848.

[6] New York's Croton Aqueduct, itself a result of the 1832 epidemic, was an exception to this generalization. Many New Yorkers, however, were not supplied with this relatively pure water. It will be recalled as well that in the medical theory of the time, the abundance and reliability of a water supply for use in street-cleaning was at least as important as its "purity" in preventing disease. For the actual developments in a number of America's larger cities, see Nelson M. Blake, *Water for the Cities: A History of the Urban Water Supply Problem in the United States* (Syracuse, 1956).

[7] *Arkansas State Democrat*, February 16, 1849. For reports of children attacked by hogs, see, for example, *Union* (St. Louis), n.d., cited in the *Illinois State Register* (Springfield), June 14, 1849; *Enquirer* (Cincinnati), August 1, 1849.

New York had grown larger, but not cleaner, in the years between 1832 and 1849. Another generation's filth had merely been added to an already impressive accumulation. No American city was dirtier.

On the morning of December 2, 1848, the "New York" rode at anchor off Staten Island. Aboard were over three hundred steerage passengers, all of whom had been exposed to cholera below decks. Prudence and public opinion alike demanded their quarantine.

But where? America's greatest port possessed no facilities adequate to quarantine fifty, let alone three hundred, immigrants. After fifteen years without cholera or yellow fever, New York's quarantine had become little more than an administrative gesture. Only the customs warehouses were large enough to accommodate so many people, and these were hurriedly converted into barrack-like hospital wards.

Such improvisations were small improvement over the holds of the "New York." Before the New Year, sixty of the immigrants had fallen ill; more than thirty had died. And over half of those originally quarantined had, as the health officer put it, "eloped," scaling the walls and making for New York or New Jersey in small boats.[8] Within a week, cases began to appear in New York City itself, in the most crowded and dirty of the immigrant boardinghouses.

Apprehensive interest turned suddenly to alarm, for it seemed that New York, like Moscow, might be scourged by cholera despite the cold of winter. Newspapers that printed cholera remedies were sold out within hours of publication. Both the New York Academy of Medicine and the Board of Health held special meetings within twenty-four hours of the discovery of the first cases. While the Academy of Medicine spent most of its time condemning the incompetence of the board, the board authorized the mayor to take whatever steps should be necessary to have the streets cleaned. A committee

8 Sterling, *op. cit.*, III, 10–13, 25.

was also chosen to arrange for the establishment of cholera hospitals.[9]

For the moment these hospitals were not needed. The bitter cold of January brought the city a momentary reprieve, and there were no more new cases. For most New Yorkers, gold fever quickly replaced fears of cholera. But the more thoughtful realized that their city enjoyed only a respite. The warmth of the coming spring would certainly quicken the dormant seeds of the disease.

New York had been fortunate in her freezing temperatures; the South was not so favored. On the sixth and eighth of December, vessels from Hamburg and Bremen brought cholera to New Orleans. In the mild New Orleans December, the disease spread rapidly among the unwashed and weary immigrants. These new arrivals quickly fanned out from New Orleans, and carried cholera with them to steamboat landings along the Mississippi, the Arkansas, and the Tennessee.[10]

Winter temperatures limited the disease to the lower South. Few doubted, however, that spring and the opening of navigation would spread cholera throughout the Mississippi Valley. Quarantines had proved themselves useless; cleanliness alone seemed to offer protection. City councils and local health boards were urged to have streets and houses cleaned and limed. "Another spring will bring the cholera among us," warned a Milwaukee editor, "sweeping like the Angel of Death over our firesides."[11]

Twenty Orange Street was not one of New York's fashionable addresses. Thirty yards from the front door was the Five Points, a focus of infection during the 1832 cholera

[9] New York City Board of Health, Minutes (hereinafter cited as Minutes), December 8, 1848, Municipal Archives and Records Center (hereinafter cited as MARC); *Evening Post* (New York), December 7, 1848.

[10] E. D. Fenner, "Report on Epidemic Cholera in the City of New Orleans . . . ," *Southern Medical Reports*, I (1849), 128–31; *Weekly Picayune* (New Orleans), January 8, 1849.

[11] *Weekly Wisconsin* (Milwaukee), December 27, 1848.

epidemic, and still the most filthy and dangerous crossroads of a rough and sprawling port. A tenement two doors up from 20 Orange Street housed one hundred and six hogs.

The poor and the criminal lived in Orange Street, and of these, only the most miserable tenanted its dark and oozing cellars. In the spring of 1849, James Gilligan, a laborer when he worked, lived with four women in a room ten or twelve feet square in the rear basement of 20 Orange Street. The door had fallen from its hinges; the sashes of its two small windows were empty. There was no bed, no chair or table— with the exception of two empty barrels, no movable furniture at all. Across these barrels the door was laid. This served as a table, and from it the five tenants ate the spoiled ham purchased at two or three cents a pound which was their usual fare.

Gilligan became ill on Friday, May 11. A habitual drinker, he thought little of his persistent cramps and vomiting. And by Saturday he felt better. On Monday the fourteenth, a local physician was notified that two of the women living in the cellar with Gilligan had sickened as well, complaining of severe cramps, vomiting, and diarrhea. Early Monday morning, Dr. Herriot made his way through the airless back yard which provided the only access to the rear basement of 20 Orange Street, lowered his head, and stepped down into the cellar. When his eyes had become accustomed to the dark, a scene macabre even for the Five Points confronted him. Three bodies, one male and two female, lay on the floor, a few rags separating them from the decaying earthen floor. Two of the three died before evening. By this time, another woman in the cellar had been taken ill, and she too died before morning.[12]

[12] The preceding account is drawn from the following sources: *Report of Seth Geer, M.D., Resident Physician of the City of New York* (New York, 1849), p. 1; *New York Journal of Medicine*, III (1849), 96; William P. Buel, "Remarks on the Asiatic Cholera in the City of New York in 1848–9," *ibid.*, IV (1850), 11–12; *Evening Post* (New York), May 17, 1849; *Tribune* (New York), May 17, 1849.

Dr. Seth Geer, the city's resident physician, was notified early that morning. It was clear to him after he had visited 20 Orange Street—as clear as it had been to Dr. Herriot—that these unfortunates had died of cholera. And so he reported to the Board of Health. This was the fifteenth of May.

Most New Yorkers were not overly alarmed. It did not seem surprising to those more comfortably situated that such wretches should die "like rotten sheep." Degraded by rum and breathing impure air, they would have succumbed had cholera never existed. Testy old Philip Hone noted on Saturday the nineteenth that the cases thus far reported had all been in Orange Street, "where water never was used internally or externally, and the pigs were contaminated by the contact of the children."[13]

The Board of Health was in a quandary. Despite intermittent efforts beginning in December, the board had not, by May, been able to establish even one cholera hospital. Fear and avarice had made it almost impossible to rent any sort of building. In desperation, Bedloe's Island, even steamboats and barges had been suggested as possible hospitals. But shipowners had proved as intractable as landlords: barges as well as houses would be permanently tainted in the public mind by their temporary use as cholera hospitals. By May, after five months of search, the only building which the board could confidently rely upon was the colored public school—and this prospective hospital possessed no sanitary facilities, not even facilities to heat water.[14] On May 16, the day after hearing the report from Orange Street, the board established its first

[13] Diary of Philip Hone, May 19, 1849, Manuscript Division, New York Historical Society.

[14] Minutes, June 2, 1849; Report of the Special Committee on Procuring Hospitals, Minutes, May 4, 1849. E. D. Morgan, chairman of the Hospital Committee, reported later that "whenever or wherever your Committee have made efforts to procure private property, that moment the alarm has been sounded, and they have been either entirely refused, or a price named, so exorbitant that it could not be entertained." New York City Board of Education, *Report . . . in Relation to the Use of Public School Houses for Hospital Purposes* (New York, 1849), p. 5.

cholera hospital. It was the second floor of a tavern and ordinarily used for meetings and militia drills. Even this crude loft was obtained only at an exorbitant rent and after a mob, threatening to burn down the building, had been dispersed.[15]

Before the epidemic had run its course, four of the city's public schools had been converted into makeshift hospitals, their desks ripped out and replaced by cots. But even these quasi-public buildings were not acquired without a struggle. The stigma of having once served as a cholera hospital could never be erased, trustees and teachers argued, while the children cast abruptly into the streets would lose interest in school and be exposed to the temptations of idleness and vile companions. They would serve only to increase the number of those susceptible to cholera.[16]

The disease soon spread from the Five Points. Alarmed New Yorkers demanded that the Board of Health contain the disease before it invaded every part of the city. And by the end of June, the Board of Health had enacted what seemed to be a comprehensive anticholera program. The alderman and assistant alderman of each ward were authorized to hire four inspectors to help enforce the health ordinances—at a salary not to exceed two dollars a day. The sale of fruits, vegetables, and fish from open carts was forbidden; and owners of filthy tenements were ordered to have them cleaned immediately.[17]

At a hastily convened meeting on the sixteenth of May, the Board of Health chose a special Sanatory Committee, which was to meet daily and direct the city's campaign against cholera. This committee, chosen from among the members of the

15 *Tribune* (New York), May 18, 19, 1849. During the course of the epidemic, 1,901 persons were admitted to New York's cholera hospitals, of whom 1,021 died. *Report of Seth Geer, M.D. . . .* , p. 12.

16 See, for example, Committee of the Teachers' Association, Memorial to the Board of Health, June 18, 1849, City Clerks' Papers, File Drawer U-60, MARC.

17 Minutes, May 16, 1849; Sanatory Committee of the Board of Health, Minutes, June 24, June 30, 1849, City Clerk's Papers, MARC.

Board of Health, was invested with the board's full powers.[18]
The committee's first act was to appoint three prominent local
physicians as medical councilors. Like the seven members of
the Special Medical Council appointed in 1832, these three
physicians had had no previous connection with the Board of
Health. Their recommendations too were reminiscent of New
York's earlier struggle with cholera. (Dr. Joseph M. Smith,
chairman of the medical advisers, drew up a broadside summarizing his admonitions to the public. Aside from a few
verbal changes, it was identical with the recommendations of
the Board of Health during the 1832 epidemic.[19])

Still the disease spread.[20] By June, many New Yorkers had
deserted their homes for the pure air of the countryside.
Those remaining provided themselves with calomel, laudanum, or perhaps those newer cholera remedies, sulphur pills
and camphor "segars." Others turned to God. Catholics who
had lived for years in mortal sin appeared again at Communion, and many of the city's Protestant churches held
regular prayer meetings. June 28 had been set aside as a day
of fasting and prayer by the General Synod of the Dutch Reform Church and the General Association of the Old School
Presbyterians.[21]

To the sorrow of clergymen, however, most New Yorkers
seemed unmoved by this threatened judgment. "How small is
the moral impression made upon the masses!" lamented one

[18] Sanatory Committee, Minutes, May 17, 31, 1849. This committee was
similar in structure and function to the Executive Committee of the Board
of Health, which functioned during the cholera epidemic seventeen years
earlier.

[19] Ten thousand copies of the broadside were printed and either posted or
distributed by policemen. Sanatory Committee, Minutes, May 17, 1849. It is
clear from the wording of the recommendations that Dr. Smith must either
have copied them or else had a very good memory of events seventeen years
earlier.

[20] It is likely that cholera's much slower spread in 1849—as compared to
1832—was due to the availability of Croton water in 1849, water not contaminated as easily as had been the shallow wells of New York in 1832.

[21] *Freeman's Journal* (New York), June 30, 1849; *Independent* (New York),
June 28, 1849.

minister. The theaters "and other places of amusement and carnal pleasure," were "in full blast." The Sabbath itself was profaned by the illicit operations of over thirty-five hundred grogshops.[22]

It seemed inevitable that the mid-summer heat would force into luxuriant growth the already well-established rootings of the disease. (Even the air seemed to have lost its elasticity, one observer noted—as it had done in the summer of 1832.) And, editorialists commented acidly, there was little chance of cholera subsiding while the streets of New York were still covered with filth and garbage.[23]

Such fears were soon justified. In July, the case rate began steadily and abruptly to rise. A week after the Fourth, eighty-five new cases and thirty deaths were reported. The weather too had grown steadily warmer, and business declined as New Yorkers left and provincial merchants feared to enter the plague-ridden city. By the fourteenth of July, only one theater remained open. At least two dozen churches had, before the month ended, closed their doors as well.

Though deaths increased, the city's streets were still filthy, still patrolled by pigs and dogs. Garbage still encrusted cellars and yards. It seemed clear that the city fathers were either ignorant or incompetent. As early as May 25, William Cullen Bryant's *Evening Post* had charged the municipal authorities with criminal neglect. The *Herald* too was quick to attack the "culpable neglect and imbecility" of the Board of Health.[24]

Nor were such attacks unjustified. Things simply did not get done—despite the statutory power of the Board of Health

---

[22] *Christian Observer* (Philadelphia), June 25, 1849; *Christian Advocate* (New York), June 7, 1849.

[23] Diary of Philip Hone, May 30, 1849, Manuscript Division, New York Historical Society; *Inquirer* (Hempstead, N.Y.), June 2, 1849.

[24] *Herald* (New York), July 9, 1849. Exacerbating such resentment was the endemic popular dislike of the medical profession, of which the Sanatory Committee seemed to have become the tool.

"to do or cause to be done *any thing* which in their opinion may be proper to preserve the health of the city."[25] The members of the Common Council who constituted the Board of Health were ill-prepared to implement such wide and ill-defined powers. Precedent and traditional penury determined that so vague a grant of power would be construed in the narrowest of fashions. New York aldermen were, moreover, notoriously immune to the promptings of civic morality. (A sardonic journalist suggested that the only way to have the city cleaned was to raise a fund and bribe the city councilmen —the standard procedure for getting things done in New York.[26] Even when the harried councilmen did attempt to enforce a regimen of strict cleanliness, they met with continual obstruction. Conflicts arose between city and state authorities, between the Board of Health and the Commissioners of the Alms-House, between the board and the president of the Croton Water Board.[27] Equally discouraging was the recalcitrant attitude of the average householder. In an admission of impotence, the Board of Health finally resorted, as it had seventeen years earlier, to requesting the city's clergymen to urge upon their congregations the sanitary regulations which the board had shown itself unable to enforce.[28] Even the best of efforts, however, could not have overcome the inertia of generations.

Nowhere was the inadequacy of traditional practice more

[25] Henry Davies, Corporation Counsel, to James Kelly, Chairman of the Sanatory Committee, City Clerk's Papers, File Drawer U-60, MARC.

[26] *Day-Book* (New York), December 8, 1848.

[27] *Sun* (New York), May 23, 1849; Christopher Morgan to Simeon Draper, May 17, 1849, City Clerks' Papers, File Drawer U-60, MARC. Croton water for cleaning the Five Points was, for example, used over the objections of the president of the Croton Water Board, who claimed that the reservoirs were too low to allow any water to be used for such a purpose. *Tribune* (New York), May 19, 1849.

[28] New York City Board of Health, *Report of the Proceedings of the Sanatory Committee . . . in Relation to the Cholera . . .* (New York, 1849), p. 32.

apparent than in the contract system of street cleaning.[29] The contracts were political manna and it was assumed that the contractor would make no more than token efforts to fulfil the duties which he had agreed to perform. When during the cholera epidemic several of the contractors were forced to actually clean the streets, they begged to be released from their contracts, pleading that they could not fulfil them without incurring grave financial loss.[30] A few contractors finally began to clean their appointed streets, but only after repeated threats. When the dirt was finally rooted up from streets and yards, it often lay uncollected for days or weeks in foul-smelling hillocks, seemingly more malignant than the same garbage or excrement left undisturbed. If gathered at all, such filth was dumped from the ends of city piers, frequently in places inaccessible to the swift tides of the river, where it lay impeding navigation and tainting the atmosphere. And it was no easy task to hire men for this dirty and unpopular work. Local hoodlums regularly stoned night-soil gatherers and sometimes shot their horses.[31] Such arrangements were a permanent menace to the health of New York's half-million inhabitants.

The city seemed unable even to bury its own dead. Bodies might lie for hours, in some cases for days, in the streets before they were started on their way to Potter's Field. After being unloaded from the scows that brought them to the city cemetery on Randall's Island, the dead were deposited in a wide trench some hundred yards in length, one body on top of another to within a foot or two of the surface. Fortunately,

29 At the risk of seeming obvious—and redundant—let me remark that in the light of contemporary medical opinion, there was no prophylactic measure more important than that of cleaning the streets. The effectiveness of public health measures can be judged only in relation to the assumptions of contemporary medical thought, not in the light of twentieth-century medical knowledge.

30 For example, see Petition of John Brady for Release from Cleaning Streets, June 23, 1849, Filed Papers of the Common Council, File Drawer U-30, MARC.

31 *Sun* (New York), May 24, 1849.

they were not allowed to lie thus and infect the city with the odor of their putrefaction. Thousands of rats swam each day from the city to the island, burrowed quickly into the hastily covered trenches, and disposed of the excess flesh before it could mortify. Within the city itself land was at a premium, and churchyards permitted the burial of coffins two and three deep.[32] Human bodies were not as numerous as the carcasses of the animals butchered each day in the city's abattoirs. During the epidemic, the bone-boiling establishments that normally disposed of these carcasses were ordered closed as menaces to the public health. As a result, the bones and offal of hundreds of animals were thrown each day into the river to putrefy, wedged against docks and slips by the returning tides.[33]

Tempering the disgraceful with the absurd was the Sanatory Committee's campaign against the city's pigs. Despite the warnings of physicians, it was almost impossible to separate the poor from their pigs, a cheap and reliable source of garbage-fattened bacon and hams. Riots and subterfuge confronted the police when they attempted to move the hogs into the city's less crowded upper wards. The porkers had to be flushed out of cellars and garrets, where their fond owners had secreted them. Nevertheless, as a result of police persistence—and clubs—five or six thousand swine were being "boarded out" by the middle of June. But concentrated now in the northern wards, they soon became a menace to the residents of these usually peaceful environs.[34]

[32] *Sun* (New York), July 20, 1849; *Evening Post* (New York), July 31, August 4, 1849; "Gothamite," *Federal Union* (Milledgeville, Ga.), August 14, 1849; Memorial to the Common Council to Prohibit Burials in Stilwell's Burial Ground . . . , July 30, 1849, Filed Papers of the Common Council, File Drawer U-81, MARC; *Sunday Dispatch* (New York), August 5, 1849.

[33] New York City Inspector, *Annual Report . . . during the Year 1849* (New York, 1850), p. 509.

[34] Horace Greeley to James W. Beekman, August 8, 1849, Beekman Family Papers, Manuscript Division, New York Historical Society; *Sun* (New York), May 22, 25, June 16, 1849; *Evening Post* (New York), May 21, 1849; Sanatory Committee, Minutes, July 13, 1849.

Despite such laudable efforts, the epidemic increased. By the end of July, business had almost ceased: hotels were empty; railroads and steamships arrived without passengers. The city's petty traders despaired, for many relied upon the custom of the provincial merchants who crowded into the city during ordinary summers. Local customers too had left the city and many small enterprisers were hard pressed to pay rents and buy fall goods. Few businessmen, however, went hungry. There were others who did; the working people were the most severely affected by the epidemic, unprepared as they were to undergo a protracted period of unemployment.

Fortunately, the disease declined rapidly. The Centre Street Cholera Hospital had been closed and Niblo's Gardens reopened by the first of August. Two weeks later, businessmen were beginning to arrive in the city, and hotels and boarding-houses lost their desolate look. Boxes and bales again blocked sidewalks and carts filled the narrow streets, while newspapers felt called upon to attack the "reprehensible" cholera reports which the Board of Health continued obstinately to issue.

Five thousand and seventeen New Yorkers had died since May 16.[35] And New York was lucky—other cities did not so easily escape.

April had been cruel, breeding cholera in dozens of American cities and villages. River and lake steamers sowed the disease at scores of landings, while the railroads, which already crisscrossed the Northwest, discharged cholera at points even more remote. The pestilence often flared up among immigrant barge and steamboat passengers, debilitated by long sea voyages, hungry, dirty, and huddled together on decks so crowded that even the sick could not lie down. Armed men

---

[35] New York City Board of Health, *Report of the Proceedings of the Sanatory Committee* . . . (New York, 1849), p. 57. A chart on this page summarizing mortality statistics for 1848 and 1849 shows by the great increase in the latter year of deaths from such diseases as dysentery, "diarrhea," cholera infantum, and the like, that many others died of cholera, though they were not diagnosed as such.

discouraged attempts to land and bury the cholera dead. Bodies were lowered unceremoniously overboard, and drifted ominously past river and lake towns.

Gold-seekers carried the disease with them across a continent. Cholera waited in brackish streams and water holes, left by one party, to be passed on to the next group following across the plains. The route westward was marked with wooden crosses and stone cairns, the crosses often bearing only a name and the word "cholera." Nowhere could the disease have been more terrifying than on these trails, where men died without physicians, without ministers, and without friends.[36]

By May, the disease had appeared as far north as Kenosha, Wisconsin. In hundreds of towns and cities, the outbreak of the first cholera case was expected daily. Newspapers in the smallest and most remote of communities were filled with demands for cleanliness, for the banishment of pigs, and for the establishment of hospitals. Managers of New England cotton mills distributed cholera tracts to their employees. Milwaukee built special bathhouses for arriving immigrants, while other town councils distributed chloride of lime to the poor.[37]

It was in the infant cities of the West, with no adequate water supply, primitive sanitation, and crowded with a transient population, that the disease was most severe. St. Louis lost a tenth of her population. Cincinnati suffered almost as severely, Sandusky even more severely than St. Louis. Sextons, undertakers, even the horses in St. Louis were exhausted in the Sisyphean task of removing and burying the dead. Carts and furniture wagons served as makeshift hearses, and many

[36] A sizable proportion of the incredibly large number of diaries and journals kept by Forty-Niners contain references to cholera. "Diseases, Drugs, and Doctors on the Oregon-California Trail in the Gold-Rush Years," an article by Georgia Willis Read (*Missouri Hist. Rev.*, XXXVIII [1944], 260–76) contains many useful references to cholera and its treatment.

[37] In some cities, the disease persisted throughout the winter, becoming epidemic in the heat of the summer. In St. Louis, there were 38 cholera deaths in January, 20 in February, 68 in March, 131 in April, and 517 in May. William M. McPheeters, *op. cit.*, p. 100.

of the dead came finally to an informal rest in the woods or on Mississippi sand bars. In Sandusky, rough unfinished boards nailed hastily together served as coffins. Even such crude amenities were unavailable in San Antonio: here, in some cases, the dead were strapped to dried oxhides and dragged along on them, livid and purple, to their graves.[38]

Few towns were sufficiently small or isolated to escape. Madison, Indiana, suffered eight to fifteen deaths a day for several weeks. In Washington, another Indiana town, there were sixty deaths among the few hundred who had not fled. At the height of the epidemic, Belleville, Illinois, had twenty new cases a day. Every store closed; business ceased, and smoke from bonfires lit to purify the air continually shrouded the town. Of three hundred and fifty persons at the camp of the United States Eighth Regiment, at Lavacca, Texas, one hundred and fifty died. In the Rio Grande Valley as a whole, an army surgeon estimated that two thousand out of twenty thousand inhabitants had succumbed. It was calculated that the southern states had lost ten thousand slaves alone, and by September the price of Negroes had already risen in response.[39]

There was little that could be done. Municipal health boards found their rudimentary powers insufficient to prevent or mitigate the epidemic. Indeed, many towns possessed no health board; in a greater number they existed more in statute than reality—except during epidemics. New York, like most states, had no public health legislation. The law providing for local boards of health, passed as an emergency cholera measure

38 *Medical News and Library*, VII (1849), 65; Patrick I. Nixon, *A Century of Medicine in San Antonio* (San Antonio, 1936), p. 97; *Daily True Democrat* (Cleveland), July 30, 31, 1849.

39 J. G. Marshall to Caleb B. Smith, June 28, 1849, R. A. Clements to Caleb B. Smith, July 21, 1849, Caleb Blood Smith Papers, Manuscript Division, Library of Congress; Gustave Koerner, *Memoirs* (Cedar Rapids, Ia., 1909), I, 543–44; N. S. Jarvis, "Report on the Rise, Progress and Decline of Epidemic Cholera in the Valley of the Rio Grande," *Southern Medical Reports*, I (1849), 438–39. Northerners opposed to slavery feared that the immediate effect of the epidemic had been to raise the price of slaves and hence prolong the existence of slavery. Cf. *Evangelist* (New York), October 11, 1849.

in June, 1832, had expired by limitation the following year.[40]
It took more than good intentions to clean a town or city; and
cleanliness, physicians agreed, was the only guarantee of immunity from cholera.

Even the largest cities lacked administrative tools. Attempts
to effect sanitary reforms were in many cities, as in New
York, paralyzed by the politically expedient contract system.
In Baltimore, a local physician remarked, the only effectual
scavenger was a heavy shower. Not even Boston, well-
governed by standards of the time, was able to thoroughly
clean its narrow and ill-graded courts, lanes, and alleys. The
filth disinterred from cellars and cesspools was piled in streets
or dumped in rivers—and, to the horror of a Boston railroad
man, on his tracks. Despite the menace of cholera, many communities were unwilling or unable to enact coercive legislation and to force citizens to clean their property. In Vincennes, householders were "earnestly urged," in Galena "earnestly requested," to clean and lime their premises. In even
the most authoritarian of communities, the penalty for non-
observance of sanitary regulations was modest, at most a fifty-
dollar fine or thirty days in jail. And even these mild penalties
were rarely imposed.

Money too was lacking. Most Americans were unwilling to
be taxed or otherwise inconvenienced at the behest of some
health board. In a city as large as Chicago, unpaid volunteers
enforced sanitary regulations. New York, like many other
communities, entrusted city council members with much of
the responsibility for enforcing such ordinances. But, as an
early chronicler of Milwaukee commented: "human nature
predominates in an Alderman—and self-preservation is the first
law of nature."[41]

----

[40] New York State, Metropolitan Board of Health, *Annual Report . . . 1866*
(New York, 1867), Appendix "F," pp. 366–72 contains an outline, "History
of the Health Laws of the State of New York," written by George Bliss, Jr.,
counsel to the board.

[41] [Frank Flower], *History of Milwaukee, Wisconsin . . .* (Chicago, 1881),
pp. 398–99.

Such a state of things could not be tolerated. Public meetings were called, to demand, to cajole, and to organize. Ward
and district committees were chosen to aid sanitary inspectors
("Committees of Safety" they were called in New York).
Once an epidemic had begun, the sick were visited at home,
and—less frequently—nursed in hospitals by volunteers. Ordinary citizens were, even in large cities, ready if necessary to
assume the duties of a paralyzed municipal government. In St.
Louis, the Board of Health completely abdicated responsibility and was soon replaced by a twelve member "Committee
of Public Health," chosen at an open meeting. As a result of a
bitter scuffle between regular and homeopathic physicians, the
Cincinnati Board of Health, originally composed of medical
men, was replaced by one containing a lawyer, an editor, a
liquor dealer, a preacher, and a mechanic.[42] Wherever officials
had shown themselves incompetent or inefficient, editors
urged fellow townsmen to call public meetings and form their
own boards of health.

Those orphaned and made destitute had also to be cared
for. And only the most radical questioned the responsibility
of private charity for alleviating such misery. The need had
only to be made known. In dozens of cities and towns, committees of "Christian gentlemen" collected and distributed
food, clothing, money, even chloride of lime to the poor.
Churches often allied themselves with these *ad hoc* committees, holding special collections for the sick and impoverished.

One problem remained even after the epidemic had departed and business resumed its usual activity: What was to
become of the orphans? Neither private persons nor informal
committees were prepared to care permanently for these
waifs. They were usually left to the churches, and in many
cases it was the impetus of the cholera epidemic that allowed
the establishment of much needed institutions for the care of
dependent children. Such, for example, was the case in Chi-

---

[42] William M. McPheeters, *op. cit.*, 106; Thomas Carroll, "Observations
on the Asiatic Cholera, as It Appeared in Cincinnati in 1849–50," *Cincinnati
Lancet & Observer*, IX (1866), 299.

cago, Milwaukee, Sandusky, San Francisco, and St. Louis. Groups of Roman Catholics sponsored many of these orphanages, since their church possessed the trained and dedicated personnel necessary to staff and administer such institutions. (Catholics were, moreover, alarmed at the moral consequences of allowing Catholic children to be raised outside the church's influence.) Other such homes were established under secular or Protestant auspices.[43]

Hospitals were the most immediate need in cholera-stricken communities, but a need not easily filled. Few communities had either the initiative or the financial resources necessary for their establishment before cholera appeared. And even with the presence of the disease lending urgency to their efforts, boards of health found it difficult to secure buildings for use as cholera hospitals. In Philadelphia, Rochester, New York, and many other cities, the rioting of the poor and the petitions of the genteel discouraged attempts to establish such "pesthouses." Threats of arson caused more than one landlord to refuse the generous rents offered by health boards. Philadelphia, like New York, had to commandeer the public schools, rip out desks, and place cots in their stead. Indeed, the Quaker City Board of Health considered itself quite fortunate in being able to procure such large and airy buildings. In other cities, abandoned or little used hotels, taverns, or country houses were suddenly transformed into cholera hospitals.[44]

[43] James Brown, *The History of Public Assistance in Chicago, 1833 to 1893* (Chicago, 1941), pp. 34–35; Daniel T. McColgan, *A Century of Charity: The First One Hundred Years of the Society of St. Vincent de Paul in the United States* (Milwaukee, 1951), I, 124; John Rothensteiner, *History of the Archdiocese of St. Louis* ... (St. Louis, 1928), II, 21–23; Zephyrin Engelhardt, *The Missions and Missionaries of California* (San Francisco, 1915), IV, 696–97. Before such permanent arrangements were made, ward committees collected money for the maintenance of orphans and tried to find homes for them.

[44] In only a few communities, such as Buffalo and St. Louis, where the Sisters of Charity allowed their hospitals and nursing care to be used in treating cholera patients, could health authorities turn to hospitals already staffed and functioning. *Freeman's Journal* (New York), July 28, 1849; Austin Flint, *Buffalo Medical Journal*, V (1849), 319; Rothensteiner, *op. cit.*, II, 19.

Once established, the hospitals did not run themselves. Medicines, nursing, and medical care were almost always inadequate. In a New York cholera hospital, patients *in extremis* lay naked on cots, covered only with a much used sheet. To many physicians, these wards served only as convenient depositories for patients already moribund. These pesthouses were administered so poorly that even physicians called for their abolition; house to house visitation—even tent colonies— would be preferable.

In the popular mind, the cholera hospitals were cold and cheerless municipal slaughterhouses, where death was hurried by the ruthless experimentation of attending physicians. Only the poorest, the most wretched, those with no one to care for them died in cholera hospitals. No respectable family would allow even its servants to enter one. Its patients were the physically and morally abandoned, "the debased and profligate" of society.

Cholera still seemed a disease of poverty and sin; lechery, gluttony, or alcoholism could as appropriately as cholera be entered on the death certificates of its victims. The deaths of the moral, the prudent, the respectable were usually ignored. They seemed anomalous and served only to increase alarm. In New York City, the *Herald* (July 17) noted that deaths by cholera "among the respectable, *including even ladies*, have all tended to produce an uncommon sensation in this city." By 1849, the connection between cholera and vice had become almost a verbal reflex. The relationship between vice and poverty was a mental reflex even more firmly established.

VII. RELIGION, SCIENCE, AND PROGRESS

Cholera was an exercise of God's will. The pious of every sect, in 1849 as in 1832, accepted cholera as a chastisement appropriate to a nation sunk in materialism and sin. Zachary Taylor, unlike Andrew Jackson, did not hesitate to recommend a day of national prayer, fasting, and humiliation.

But beneath a traditional rhetoric of sin and retribution, the insidious conquest of a once omnipotent God by his own laws progressed apace. Cholera was retributive, but a retribution more and more autonomous, an automatic governor upon men's passions and indiscretions.

Asiatic cholera was a disease of "filth, of intemperance, and of vice." In the doctrine of predisposing causes, science and morality continued their unself-conscious liaison. The brigades of drunkards and prostitutes annihilated in 1832 were resurrected in the pious hope that a new generation might profit by their unfortunate example. Even those Americans who explicitly rejected the idea that cholera threatened only the poor and the sinful spoke of the evil effects of intemperance, of imprudence, and of sexual excess. Spiritual means could not be neglected in its prevention.

Early in July, General Taylor recommended that the first Friday in August be observed as a day of fasting, prayer, and humiliation. Mayors and governors immediately seconded the President's laudable injunction. But even before President Taylor's proclamation, the godly had been active: the General Synod of the Dutch Reformed and the General Assembly of the Presbyterian (Old School) churches had already appointed their own days of prayer. Public meetings, mayors, and city councils had recommended local fast days. In St. Louis, the Committee of Health did so.[1]

The National Fast—it fell on Friday, the third of August— was quietly observed, at least by the churchgoing portion of the community. Business was suspended; and in most towns, union meetings brought Methodists and Baptists, Episcopalians and Presbyterians together in prayer. Jewish congregations held special fast-day services, while Catholics gathered in their churches to hear the votive Mass, *Pro Tempore Pestilentia*. Even Shakers joined in imploring "the Almighty in his own good time, to stay the destroying hand."[2]

"Non-churchgoers" welcomed the fast day as another Sunday, an occasion for relaxation and, in cholera times, prophylactic tippling. A horrified observer of New York's fast day encountered a dozen men zigzagging drunkenly across his path in less than a half hour. The American Museum and theaters were crowded. Even more scandalous to evangelical Christians were the "four immense trains" furnished by the Long Island Railroad to transport a mob of rowdies to a course in Brooklyn where they watched "a trotting match between a pair of quadrupeds."[3]

The city poor seemed a race apart, as untouched by reli-

[1] See, for example, *Presbyterian Herald* (Louisville, Ky.), June 21, 1849; *Christian Intelligencer* (New York), June 14, 1849; *State Register* (Springfield, Ill.), July 5, 1849; Richard Edwards, *Edward's Great West and Her Commercial Metropolis* . . . (St. Louis, 1860), p. 408.

[2] James Prescott's Journal (kept in New Lebanon, New York), August 3, 1849, Shaker Papers, Box 23, folder 143, Manuscript Division, Library of Congress.

[3] *Christian Advocate* (New York), August 9, 1849.

gion as the savages of Burma or Senegal.[4] Of what use were fast days against cholera, questioned Bryant's *Evening Post* (June 2, 1849), when those in greatest danger were not in the habit of spending time in church? By 1849, the alarmed editorialist continued, most city churches had become social as well as religious associations of the respectable and the well to do. The poor could neither afford seats, nor "without making themselves uncomfortably conspicuous, mingle with the fashionable and wealthy who attend these churches." True, some attention was beginning to be shown. But a few city missions and free churches could exert little influence upon such masses of misery and irreligion.

Open infidelity had become a class attitude. The poorest and most apathetic ignored religion, while the most able and critical among the workers, the mechanics and artisans who could think beyond their next meal, became freethinkers, joined the Masons, Odd Fellows, or Druids.[5] They had no love for fast days.

As for this particular fast day—it was mere "political religious canting," a scheme of the orthodox to reunite Church and State. (Every such attempt, warned opponents of orthodoxy, must be vigilantly opposed; history recorded the fate of dissenters when the self-righteous Puritans ruled Massachusetts

[4] Even the traditionally unquestioning faith of the Irish had, it seemed, been weakened by their hardships in the Old and New Worlds. An Indiana priest wrote that many Irish immigrants twenty and thirty years old had never made their first communion: "They scarcely know there is a God; they are ashamed to attend Catechism and when they do come they do not understand the instruction. I am expecting help from the cholera; it is a better teacher than I." Letter of Father Hippolyte Du Pontavice, June 21, 1849, quoted by Sister Mary Carol Schroeder, *The Catholic Church in the Diocese of Vincennes, 1847–1877* ("Catholic University of America Studies in American Church History," Vol. XXXV; Washington, 1946), p. 58. Urban priests voiced similar complaints.

[5] "Open infidelity has descended to the lower ranks. . . . It now burrows in the narrow streets, and lanes, and purlieus of our large cities and towns. . . ." Robert Baird, *Religion in the United States* (Glasgow, 1844), pp. 650–51, cited in Albert Post, *Popular Freethought in America, 1825–1850* (New York, 1943), p. 32. From the content of free-thinking magazines and papers, it is apparent —as common sense tells us—that the very lowest in the social scale were not followers of any organized anticlerical movement.

Bay.) There existed no executive power which justified such action by the President. In any case, prayer and fasting would not protect man from cholera, "only a close, accurate and undeviating attention to facts." Religion, as seen by the freethinker, was but another cause of ignorance and mysticism, and hence of cholera. (Could one deny that the otherworldliness of Christianity impeded sanitary progress?) One freethinking "physician" hailed "the advent of this Cholera as the stretching forth of the strong arm of Deity, coming in aid of *liberalism* and of *mutual illumination,* to strike the death blow to superstition, popedom and priestcraft."[6] Theology was but the ignorance of natural causes reduced to a system.

There seemed to be no limit, their infidel opponents charged, to the hypocrisy and illogic of the orthodox. Evangelical Christians spent huge sums in rescuing the souls of savages in distant lands, while misery and despair increased a few hundred yards from their doors. American charity should be exercised in alleviating the condition of the nation's poor, not in evangelizing heathen incapable of understanding the meaning of Christianity. Even in cholera times, the poor and oppressed were offered prayer, not bread. But then what could be expected of genteel pewholders.

They can't clean the cellars, and the lanes—visit the hovels of the poor, the destitute, the widow, and the orphan, especially if they are sick; and more especially if they are vicious, and their sickness is the cholera. But they must do something, and what can they do but pray? This is easy. It neither soils their fine clothes, blisters their soft hands, offends their nostrils by noisome smells, nor shocks their fine sensibilities by witnessing constant instances of misery, sickness, destitution, and death.[7]

Most respectable Americans scorned such impious doctrines. They supported missionary and Bible societies and lauded their

[6] "A Physician," *Independent Beacon,* I (1849), 147. The rhetoric of the freethinkers shared much of that strangely wedded mixture of romantic and millennial fervor which informed that of their opponents, the "evangelicals."

[7] "J. L. G.," *Boston Investigator,* August 1, 1849.

Puritan fathers. When the judgments of God were abroad in the land, what, they felt, could be more appropriate than fasting and prayer.

A national fast was peculiarly appropriate. Never before, churchgoing Americans agreed, had a nation been so blessed by God. But material prosperity and spiritual enlightenment made America's sins all the more unforgivable; a pious ancestry had just cause to be disappointed in its children. The nation's sins were becoming ever more alarming.

And none were more disturbing than avarice and materialism. The mad quest after California's gold, fast-day jeremiads warned, was but an extreme instance of a covetousness so universal as to have subverted even America's churches. The United States had, as a nation, "been so bounteously blessed, that the giver is concealed . . . by the cloud of his own gifts." The fast-day proclamations of at least two governors prayed that the Lord might check this immoderate desire for wealth; if cholera demonstrated anything, it was the existence of something in the world beside business.[8] (The anxieties of business were, appropriately, themselves exciting causes of cholera. As a preventive against the disease, New York's Sanatory Committee urged that the "pursuits of gain, and the excitement of business be suspended.")[9]

In the context of traditional Christian ethics, the enterpriser occupied a peculiarly ambiguous position. To the American economy he seemed indispensable. Initiative and ambition produced material good—felling forests, constructing railroads, building great cities, and feeding and clothing their inhabitants.

[8] State of Vermont, "Proclamation, by the Governor . . . Carlos Coolidge" (Windsor, March 1, 1849), Broadsides, SY 1849-43, New York Historical Society; Commonwealth of Massachusetts, "A Proclamation for a Day of Public Fasting, Humiliation, and Prayer," March 10, 1849, Broadside Portfolio 59, No. 15, Library of Congress; *Banner of the Cross* (Boston), XI (August 11, 1849), 252. Attacks on materialism and worldliness were, of course, no novelty. In 1849, however, they were ubiquitous—as they had not been in 1832.

[9] Sanatory Committee of the Board of Health, Minutes, August 6, 1849, City Clerk's Papers, Municipal Archives and Records Center.

Ambition, on the other hand, was responsible for much misery: the helpless were oppressed, while the oppressor endangered his soul as surely as he did the bodies of those he exploited. And nine out of ten failed in mercantile endeavors. Moralists constantly warned of the practical as well as the spiritual dangers of excess ambition. "To strive for competence is a praiseworthy effort—to strive for more, is unphilosophical and unwise."[10] But many did—and lost their substance and often their souls in futile emulation of the Astors and Girards.

And worse yet, greed seemed to have become a leading determinant of national policy. Northern fast-day sermons dwelt frequently on America's recent despoliation of her helpless southern neighbor. We had acquired our Naboth's vineyard—but at the cost of much blood and gold. Even more disgraceful, in the opinion of many northern clergymen, was the continued bondage of several million Africans. Did not Scripture declare that chains should be struck off? The state was not a limited liability corporation: every American was morally responsible for its actions. Not that Americans were not culpable as individuals. Intemperance, Sabbath-breaking, and infidelity were prevalent enough, sermons accused, to provoke a judgment far harsher than cholera. (In the South, of course, the Mexican War and Negro slavery were not admissible as sins.)[11]

To the most orthodox, cholera was not simply a punishment for national and personal sins, but a punishment which proceeded directly from the hand of God. Cholera was one of the means with which Jehovah swept "with the besom of destruction nations degraded by superstition, and sift[ed] as chaff from wheat the vicious out of mixed populations." Though

10 *Olive Branch* (Boston), July 28, 1849.

11 Compare the discussions by Clayton S. Ellsworth, "American Churches and the Mexican War," *American Historical Review*, XLV (1940), 301–26, and John R. Bodo, *The Protestant Clergy and Public Issues 1812–1848* (Princeton, N.J., 1954), pp. 213–22. The present writer found the Mexican War condemned generally by northern Protestants, though vehemence varied directly with the fervency of the author's antislavery convictions.

second causes normally determined health and illness, the Christian must never forget that first causes were under the Lord's direct control. "Shall there be evil in the city and the Lord hath not done it." Cholera was clearly a divine imposition.[12]

What had science learned of it? The residents of orthodox pulpits were quick to observe that the causes of cholera remained a mystery. Indeed, it seemed to obey the laws of no other disease. "What," they asked, "but a palpable miracle could more clearly mark it as a visitation from the Most High?" Even a Philadelphia professor of medicine could offer no other explanation; only the will of the Lord, he assured his students, could account for the reappearance of a disease that had been quiescent for so many years. "Let those who smile or sneer at this solution, name a better one if they can?"[13]

Professor Mitchell seems, however, to have been almost unique among physicians in his confession of faith. Smiles and sneers, not grave agreement, were the expected reactions to his devout sentiments. More representative of medical opinion were the thousands of pages written by physicians on cholera, none of which mentioned, let alone attributed the disease to, the deity. God seemed out of place in a medical journal. Indeed, many physicians actively resented the inference that cholera was caused by some supernatural agency. "We have never sat at the council-board of the Almighty, . . . and refrain from prying into his secrets," wryly commented one practi-

[12] *Herald of the Prairies* (Chicago), July 18, 1849; *Friend's Review,* II (July 28, 1849), 713. Though the Lord might use natural means—as insects in the plague of locusts—it did not mean that these natural agencies were not set in motion by his will. "A. A.," *Observer* (New York), August 11, 1849.

[13] "A.D.," *Central Watchman* (Cincinnati), July 6, 1849; Thomas D. Mitchell, *Lecture on the Epidemic Cholera . . .* (Philadelphia, 1849), p. 7. See also, for example, on the "unnatural" nature of cholera: *Presbyterian* (New York), July 17, 1849; George Peck, *Christian Advocate* (New York), August 16, 1849; *Connecticut Courant* (Hartford), July 18, 1849; Diary of Andrew Lester, August 3, 1849, Manuscript Division, New York Historical Society; *Free Press* (Detroit), July 24, 1849; *Presbyterian Herald* (Louisville, Ky.), August 9, 1849.

tioner. After the epidemic, the president of the Wisconsin State Medical Society stated his hope

that no member of this Society . . . allowed himself to be satisfied with the reflection that the result was one of God's providence, but that he more properly attributed it to his ignorance of the nature and character of the pestilence, and that he determined not to be satisfied till he had fully unravelled the mystery.[14]

No man of science could be satisfied with supernatural explanations of natural events.

Such an attitude disturbed pious Americans. Though only a farseeing minority in the ministry had explicitly attacked science during the 1832 epidemic, by 1849 such attacks had become commonplace. Clerical polemicists depicted cholera as a direct rebuke to scientific pretensions; savants kindled fires in the streets, argued and then extinguished the fires, endorsed dozens of equally useless nostrums, and could agree upon no explanation of the disease's origin—though all were certain that it did not come from the hand of God. Alarmed clergymen warned that America had become a land of "practical atheists"; the minds of men had been directed toward second causes alone. Many Americans were well educated but without faith in God, for religion and education had been separated. "In the study of nature's laws, they have lost sight of nature's divine Author and Governor."[15] The enticements of the world and the achievements of science threatened to fill men's minds to the exclusion of all else.

The progress of natural science had indeed been overwhelming. Element after element had been discovered; the laws of health and disease seemed to be at last within man's grasp. Yet Paris, as the orthodox pointed out, the center of progress in medicine and chemistry, protected by advanced and well-en-

[14] Alfred L. Castleman, *Proceedings of the Wisconsin State Medical Society*, 1855–56, p. 34, cited in Peter T. Harstad, "Sickness and Disease on the Wisconsin Frontier" (unpublished Master's thesis, University of Wisconsin, 1959), p. 61.

[15] *Gospel Messenger* (Utica, N.Y.), August 10, 1849

forced health regulations, had been severely scourged by cholera. Hospitals and laboratories could not avert the judgments
of heaven. Albert Barnes, one of America's most influential
evangelists, declared cholera to be a visitation aimed particularly at the vanities of natural science. Christians must defend
the reality of God's special providences, for if there were no
special providence, if the Lord could not violate his established
laws, there would be no miracles. And without miracles, the
Bible would be little more than moralizing.[16]

Yet even the most orthodox accepted without question the
ultimate sufficiency of second causes. "The Almighty,"
Americans of all denominations agreed, "conducts the order
of Providence by *rule*—rules that are alike at all times and
abiding."[17] A pious churchgoer, if he should sup on oysters
and cucumbers during a cholera epidemic, could not hope to
escape on the strength of his Christian profession. As well
might he hold on to the end of a lighted fuse and expect
Providence to save him from the explosion. The law of
providence, the *Independent* (New York, October 11, 1849)
affirmed, would not act, if others were infringed by it. Even
Universalists and freethinkers would be spared, though they
were not God's chosen, should they adopt wise hygienic measures and thus bring themselves into an "external condition
analogous to that of the people of God generally, and thus
come within the line of that protecting mercy vouchsafed
them."[18]

[16] Albert Barnes, "The Pestilence," *American National Preacher*, XXIII
(1849), 196–202, 207.

[17] The quotation continues: "Who however shall set bounds to the *physical*
and the *moral*—and pretend to tell where one ends and the other begins? Who
can say whether it is from chemical or moral causes that this community is
scourged, while that is spared?" *Scioto Gazette* (Chillicothe, Ohio), August 1,
1849.

[18] For example, Mother Theodore Guerin, founder of an order of Catholic
sisters, wrote to the sisters at Madison, Indiana, March 21, 1849: "Be cheerful,
kind to one another. Have nothing on your conscience that could trouble you.
Do not fast. Let your food be wholesome and well prepared. Keep your house,
the yard, and also your persons clean. Change your linen often. . . . Finally,
my dear daughters, pray." *Journals and Letters of Mother Theodore Guerin*
. . . (St. Mary-of-the-Woods, Ind., 1937), pp. 280–81.

One sinned against the Holy Ghost, but also against the laws of health; cholera was a result of appetites undenied, but equally the result of poor drainage and ventilation. Even the orthodox ministry had begun to preach the gospel of sanitary reform. Man "had no more right to neglect the body than . . . the soul." Cholera was the product of neglecting both.

If cholera had no other mission than this, to sanction the practice of temperance and cleanliness, and to denounce the penalties against artificial and undenied appetites, and putrescent inhalations, it is yet an angel of mercy to the world, if mankind will suffer themselves to be instructed by it.[19]

Even the rhetorical strategy of the godly had been infiltrated by the prevailing empiricism. Elaborate tables demonstrated the higher percentage of mortality among the intemperate and the vicious. An Indiana minister, for example, totted up the cholera deaths in his community and concluded that they showed "a difference of fifty-five to seventeen in favor of the habits of a religious life."[20]

The orthodox position was clearly equivocal. They had conceded almost all of their opponent's assumptions and had now to argue in their terms. God's power to determine earthly happenings was no longer the central reality in men's lives, but a theoretical strong point in the struggle against infidelity. A fast day was, nevertheless, an appropriate, indeed a much-needed affirmation of the fact that America was a Christian nation.[21] It seemed fitting that Americans should pray for deliverance—though that deliverance would come only as a result of their own efforts.

To the opponents of orthodoxy, this seemed hardly a con-

[19] "E. M.," *Morning Star* (Dover, N.H.), XXIV (August 15, 1849), 69.

[20] Joseph G. Wilson, *Voice of God in the Storm* . . . (Lafayette, Ind.), p. 32 n. Hospital and board of health reports, almost without fail, recorded the proportion of the intemperate among those dying from cholera.

[21] ". . . it is another and a solemn declaration to the nation and to the world that we are a religious, a Christian nation; that christianity enters as an element into the administration of our national affairs." *Ohio Observer* (Hudson), August 1, 1849.

sistent position. No amount of prayer, fasting, and humiliation, they charged, could bring relief from an epidemic. While the chief executive wasted his and the nation's time with pious proclamations, the poor and ignorant continued in their perilous habits of life. Supplication was not enough. "Prayer, without at the same time forsaking sin and doing right, is an utter mockery, and deserves a curse. We must now cleanse and purify ourselves."[22] To Universalists and Unitarians, freethinkers and associationists, cholera was a result of injustice in society, not a judgment upon individual sins.

A fast day was at best useless, at worst a source of additional cholera cases. On the part of the President, it was a cynical gesture of political accommodation. "No one," a liberal editor commented, "can be so unwise at this day, as to suppose that a physical evil is to be removed by moral or religious means—that the Deity will neutralize the poisonous effluvia which their own ignorance or carelessness has suffered to be generated around their dwellings!"[23] Cholera, like other diseases, resulted from the violation of immutable laws. To violate such laws brought inevitable punishment—according to the "system" which it had pleased God to adopt in the moral and physical government of the world. There was no atoning blood for cholera. It was clear, at least to the most radical, that *"all evil"* resulted from the violation of natural laws. Societies as well as men might depart from nature's ordered pattern; nations like men might suffer from moral as well as physical ills.[24]

[22] Charles D. Meigs, *Remarks on Spasmodic Cholera* (Philadelphia, 1849), p. 68; William R. Alger, *Inferences from the Pestilence and the Fast . . .* (Boston, 1849), p. 11; "H. G. E.," *Christian Register*, XXVIII (August 11, 1849), 126; *Harbinger*, n.d., cited in *ibid.*, XXVIII (January 20, 1849), 9.

[23] *Weekly Echo* (New Bedford, Mass.), n.d., cited in *Liberator* (Boston), August 3, 1849.

[24] "H," *Sun* (New York), July 24, 1849; *Model Worker* (Utica, N.Y.), December 22, 1849; *Boston Investigator*, July 25, August 3, August 15, October 11, 1849; *Weekly Wisconsin* (Milwaukee), July 11, 1849; *Sunday Times* (New York), July 8, 1849; *Sunday Dispatch* (New York), December 17, 1849. The anticlerical, though not as vocal as in 1832, naturally seized upon the fast day to attack the "evangelicals." The Old School—antimission—Baptists also opposed it, because of man's presumption in making such demands. Cf. Gilbert Beebe, "The Pestilence," *Signs of the Times*, XVII (July 18, 1849), 110.

Traditional Christian metaphors of the soul's health were naturally widened to include the health or disease of a "sinful" —"unnatural"—society, while at the same time the metaphor became more specifically biological and, consequently, more and more a substantive statement, less and less clearly a metaphor. The absolute value of personal salvation was being replaced by that of nature as norm. Science, of course, rather than theology interpreted these new commandments.

The abolitionists, though by no means infidels, also opposed the fast day. They could not observe the hypocritical recommendations of a slave-driving President, observe a proclamation which seemed merely a draft upon the piety of the nation —payable in 1852. The United States could not expect immunity. Would God spare a nation cursed by human bondage which still presumptuously declared its surpassing piety? William Lloyd Garrison spent August 3 in observing the anniversary of emancipation in the West Indies; he would honor no fast appointed by a slaveholder.

But most Americans approved of the fast day as laudable in intent, if not actually efficacious. The extremism of the abolitionists was not only impious, but subversive and distasteful. (To the South, it was but another proof of northern fanaticism.) Most northerners, though deploring slavery, deplored even more strongly the extravagances of the Garrisonites. They did "more towards perpetuating slavery in this country than any other portion of our citizens."[25]

25 "Truth," *Connecticut Courant* (Hartford), August 11, 1849.

VIII. THE NATURE OF POVERTY AND THE PREVENTION OF DISEASE

To most Americans, poverty was still a moral, not a social, phenomenon—as was cholera. The vice, filth, and ignorance that bred poverty nurtured cholera as well. No longer, however, did a man's moral condition seem sufficient explanation of his immunity or susceptibility. Disease was becoming more and more a product of environment: the city and the tenement assumed leading places in the list of cholera's predisposing causes.

Not all poverty was unworthy. Nor did cholera attack the prudent and industrious workingman. The vicious poor, the drunkard and idler, the prostitute and thief, were its proper victims. The filth that surrounded these self-sentenced exiles from society mirrored accurately their inner decay; they, not "the virtuous and industrious poor," suffered disproportionately. If hard-working mechanics and artisans were stricken, most Americans believed, it was not because of their moral, but their temporal proximity to the vicious and dissolute.[1]

[1] *Religious Herald* (Richmond, Va.), September 6, 1849. The few surviving hospital statistics that report the occupations of those dying of cholera show them to have been overwhelmingly servants and laborers. Cf. New York City Board of Health, *Report of the Proceedings of the Sanatory Committee* . . . (New York, 1849), pp. 70–71, 72–73, 83, 97.

The labor of America's farmers, artisans, and mechanics had made and sustained the republic. The dignity of labor was secure in the formulas of conventional rhetoric; these "real people," these "noble men," were not society's lower classes, but rather its foundation classes. "On their foreheads and palms God has set his enduring seal of nobility, and the shifts of fashion, the voice of public opinion, and the assumptions of aristocracy can never obliterate it." Despite the disdain of the thoughtless, the mechanic in his city workshop was as indispensable to society as the farmer in his fields. And, moralists noted, St. Paul a tentmaker and Jesus a carpenter, had both been mechanics.[2]

What could be more absurd than the pretensions of America's self-proclaimed aristocrats? Almost invariably they were men whose fathers had been farmers or artisans, and whose grandchildren would most likely fill the same humble place in society. The poor man was healthier, his step more sound than the careworn man of wealth, who lived out his hectic and unnatural life far removed from God's open fields. Real poverty lay not in lack of riches, but in discontent with one's lot. America was a land of opportunity and equality, in which productive work alone conferred genuine distinction.[3]

Or was it? Far more than in 1832, newspapers, magazines, and sermons self-consciously affirmed the dignity of the worker, deplored the pretensions and cares of wealth. The assumptions of Jacksonian rhetoric had become explicitly homiletic: exhortation replaced effusion as the divergence between image and reality in American society became increasingly disturbing.

2 "Facts for Mechanics," *Morning Star*, XXIV (August 8, 1849), 68; *Sun* (New York), December 7, 1848; *Organ* (New York), December 9, 1848, p. 189; *Herald of the Prairies* (Chicago), January 17, 1849; *Cumberland Valley Sentinel* (Chambersburg, Pa.), December 25, 1849; George C. Foster, *New York in Slices* (New York, 1849), pp. 4–5; *Brownlow's Whig* (Knoxville, Tenn.), September 29, 1849.

3 *People's Friend* (Covington, Ind.), August 25, 1849; *Gazette* (Vincennes, Ind.), May 31, 1849; *Sun* (New York), June 13, 1849; *Ohio Observer* (Hudson), December 13, 1848; *Gazette* (St. Joseph, Mo.), July 20, 1849.

In the categories of popular thought, the vicious were easily distinguished from the industrious poor. In practice, this was not so easily accomplished. The hard-working mechanic was likely to spend much of his wages on drink, was often, if involuntarily, unemployed, failed to attend church, and lived in crowded and filthy tenements. To respectable, servant-employing, churchgoing Americans, the city poor were a uniformly unappetizing group.

Americans were not surprised that such degraded souls should succumb to cholera. And despite bitter experience to the contrary, it was believed not only that the lower orders suffered severely from the disease, but that they suffered almost to the exclusion of the better sort.[4] Cholera among the respectable was, as in 1832, attributed to hidden vice or unaccustomed imprudence.

Famine and revolution in Europe crowded American cities with newly arrived immigrants. Poor, ignorant, friendless, and often unaccustomed to city life, they tenanted the dirtiest boarding houses and the most decayed tenements. They were the first to be attacked by cholera.

More than 40 per cent of those dying of cholera in New York had been born in Ireland. The cities with the greatest immigrant populations—St. Louis, Cincinnati, New York, New Orleans—were those which suffered most severely during the epidemic.[5] The decimation of St. Louis and Cincinnati

---

[4] Belief in personal misconduct as a cause of disease did not die easily, despite any amount of evidence to the contrary—for it was "a great consolation." Charles Anderson to Caleb B. Smith, July 3, 1849, Caleb Smith Papers, Manuscript Division, Library of Congress.
The dichotomy between the deserving and the vicious poor was well-nigh universal in nineteenth-century thought. Karl Marx's distinction between the "proletariat" and the "lumpen-proletariat" is simply another reflection of this pervasive assumption.

[5] At the height of the epidemic in St. Louis, 1,182, or about four-fifths of the 1,556 who died, were Catholic. John Rothensteiner, History of the Archdiocese of St. Louis . . . (St. Louis, 1928), II, 18. A tabulation of hospital statistics from six cities (Cincinnati, New York, Buffalo, Brooklyn, Boston, and New Orleans) shows that 4,309 of 5,301 patients whose place of birth was

seemed, at least to some Americans, to be more attributable to the drinking and Sabbath-breaking of newly arrived immigrants than to any lack of sanitation in the cities themselves. Philip Hone agreed completely. The immigrants were, he noted in his diary,

filthy, intemperate, unused to the comforts of life, and regardless of its proprieties . . . flock to the populous towns of the great west, with disease engendered on Shipboard, and increased by bad habits on shore, they inoculate the inhabitants of these beautiful Cities, and every paper we open is only a record of premature mortality.[6]

Cholera was an acute phase of a chronic malady; immigration had become a permanent threat to American institutions. Even in normal times, "degraded foreigners" populated almshouses and hospitals.[7] At election time, immigrant votes were sold to the highest bidder, while each week the Sabbath was profaned by their whiskey-drinking and carousing. How long, questioned a Congregational weekly, would our remaining Puritanism survive this process of dilution? Someday, these new citizens and their children would be as loud in asserting themselves as those Americans whose ancestors had landed at Plymouth Rock or Jamestown. But would they be fitted for such privileges? Only unceasing missionary activity among

---

known were born outside the United States. This tabulation of hospital statistics is based on published board of health and hospital reports. Since these are hospital statistics and since people of the "better sort" did not go to hospitals, these figures do not accurately reflect the absolute percentage of immigrants succumbing to cholera, though they do reflect clearly the low economic status of the newly arrived immigrant.

6 Diary of Philip Hone, June 30, 1849, Manuscript Division, New York Historical Society. Americans were especially shocked at the German diet of green vegetables, sauerkraut, and strong beer—a diet which seemed to invite cholera.

7 Many journalists and ordinary citizens were disturbed by the threat of immigration to the public health. "The bodies of the miserable outcasts are charged with infection on the voyage, and then they are turned loose here to spread ship fever, or whatever contagious disease they may have imbibed, or to occupy the fever wards of our hospitals to the exclusion of our own citizens." Sunday Times (New York), March 11, 1849.

them, pious Americans were warned, would assure their virtue and good citizenship.[8]

Americans had always thought of their country as an "asylum for the poor, virtuous, and oppressed of other lands." But the founding fathers could never have foreseen that the deserving poor of an earlier day would have, in less than a century, become the degraded and criminal refuse that polluted American shores in 1849. Few Americans, even the most moderate, could deny that "a very large proportion of the foreigners that have come to this country for several years past are vicious and worthless." A victim in the Old World of too much law and too much restraint, the immigrant could not, it seemed, conceive of responsible citizenship or ordered liberty. In minds long fettered, liberty too often meant license and freedom irresponsibility.[9] The votes of foreigners already decided elections in New York, Pittsburgh, St. Louis, and other cities. Nativists warned that these foreigners would soon have "control of the ballot box; and when they [did], mobocracy would be the order of the day."[10]

The Irish presented the greatest menace. Even the Germans, with their beer-drinking, their freethought, and their Continental Sunday were not as great a threat to American institutions. That the Irish suffered severely from cholera was but additional testimony to their ignorance, their habitual filth and drunkenness; Irish wakes denied propriety even to death. Prosperous Americans knew Irish men and women only as servants, and as servants who often remained as strangers though living under the same roof. An Irish peasant, working in a well-scrubbed Protestant kitchen must have often seemed to his masters dirty, resentful, wilful, and invincibly ignorant.

[8] *Christian Mirror* (Portland, Me.), February 1, 1849. The pious deplored especially the role of immigrants as whiskey-sellers and consumers. They had, it seemed, "not been accustomed in their native lands to regard the business as disreputable." *Watchman and Observer* (Richmond, Va.), March 22, 1849; *Central Watchman* (Cincinnati), September 28, 1849.

[9] *Western Eagle* (Cape Girardeau, Mo.), August 3, 1849.

[10] "R," *Christian Register* (Boston), XXVIII (April 14, 1849), 59.

He was, moreover, the stubbornest kind of Catholic. They are, in the words of an alarmed New York minister,

Catholics to the back-bone: an Irishman as part of his religion must not eat meat on Friday; he must run loose all of the Sabbath, and also every evening of the week, and he must be allowed to deceive and lie, even when truth would answer his purpose better.[11]

At best, the devoted Catholic was to be pitied as a priest-ridden worshipper of the Beast. Evangelical ministers still assured their flocks that the Church of Rome was the Whore of Babylon, the Mother of Harlots foretold in Revelation. Nevertheless, only a few Protestant divines went so far as to interpret cholera as a deserved visitation upon the Catholics.[12] Those that did blamed the priests for the death of their parishioners. Had they not granted these poor helots a general absolution? And had this not been followed by the drinking and reveling which brought death?

Many Americans were prepared to pity the ragged and untutored Irishman, but not even the most understanding could condone the "cynical machinations" of the Catholic hierarchy (a position similar to that of many twentieth-century liberals who find this distinction a convenient compromise between liberalism and vulgar anti-Romanism). While his clergy labored among the dying in New York, Bishop Hughes was, according to James Gordon Bennett's *Herald* (August 8, 1849), luxuriating in the safety of Saratoga Springs. Dramatizing to most Americans the hierarchical and antidemocratic nature of the Roman church was the collection of Peter's Pence during the summer of 1849 for use in maintaining the temporal power and defeating the Roman republicans. It seemed strange that American citizens should help preserve arbitrary government,

11 John Todd, "Christian Duties to Domestics," *Evangelist* (New York), July 26, 1849. Reverend Todd suggested that domestics be required to save a portion of their salary as a condition of their employment, that they be urged to attend family worship, and that they be forced to eat meat on Fridays.

12 "Criticus," *Christian Advocate* (New York), July 12, 1849; *Nonpareil* (Cincinnati), n.d., cited in the *Pilot* (Boston), August 25, 1849.

that their dollars should purchase the bullets with which patriots and republicans were slain.

The church did make concessions. For Catholics to be accepted as Americans like any others, they must conform to the moral precepts of American Protestantism. Thus, for example, in an effort to avert cholera, the Cincinnati *Catholic Telegraph* participated wholeheartedly in a campaign to encourage temperance and a stricter observation of the Sabbath. Nor, Catholic editorialists commented, were the Irish as ruffianly and ungovernable as their critics would have them. On the contrary, because of their Catholic habits of mind, they were "contented with their position and state of life."[13]

Not all accusations during the epidemic were made by Protestants. Catholics were quick to boast of the fidelity of their clergy—and to make pointed comparisons with those Protestant shepherds who had deserted their flocks. Many Catholics, they charged as well, were denied the consolations of religion in almshouses and hospitals by the "long-faced psalm singing bigots" superintending these institutions.[14]

The devotion of the Catholic clergy, and especially the Sisters of Charity, won the often reluctant praise of their Protestant neighbors. As Richard Henry Dana wrote to his orthodox and intolerant wife: "In spite of all you say, I believe that if anybody goes to Heaven from Boston it will be the Sisters of Charity and the Roman Catholic clergy."[15] Admiration of the

[13] *Catholic Telegraph*, May 10, 1849; *Freeman's Journal* (New York), March 24, 1849. This appeal showed how far at least one Catholic publicist misjudged the American temper. A defense of the Irish as being "contented" served only to reinforce the contentions of those who attacked the traditional tyranny of the church. It was the reputed personal pugnaciousness of the Irish, not any political activism, which Americans found most distasteful.

[14] *Catholic Telegraph* (Cincinnati), July 12, 1849.

[15] R. H. Dana to Mrs. Dana, August 11, 1849, Dana Papers, Massachusetts Historical Society. For other praise of Catholic benevolence, see, for example, *State Register* (Springfield, Ill.), August 16, 1849; Boston Board of Health, *Report on Asiatic Cholera* . . . (Boston, 1849), p. 24; W. T. Hamilton, "Cholera in New Orleans," *Alabama Planter* (Mobile), January 1, 1849; *True Whig* (Nashville, Tenn.), August 24, 1849; *Sunday Times* (New York), December 3, 1848.

Sisters was general and unqualified; their benevolence was of a practical sort, their lives not idled away in the convent's living tomb.

The Jews, like the Irish, were part of an urban America. But as was not true of resentment against the Irish, hostility toward the Jews was tempered by a peculiarly American ambivalence. Unresolved tensions in American life were faithfully mirrored in the contradictory, even paradoxical, image assigned to the Jew. He, like the American, was a pious Shylock, a venturesome conservative, an individualistic traditionalist. To reject him completely was to reject much that was American.[16]

It was also to reject Christ. For the Jews occupied a peculiar place in the chiliasm of pious Americans. Often contemptible, even loathsome, as individuals, the Jews had as a race been preserved for some great purpose. Their misery, persecution, and degradation bore witness to the fate of those who rejected Christ. Only the millennium would bring their conversion. "Their miraculous preservation is a standing proof of the verity of our holy oracles; and many of the glorious prophecies of the Bible are yet to be fulfilled by their restoration to national greatness, and God's favor."[17] The condition of the Jews was a carefully observed index to the proximity of the millennium.

America's cities were no longer American; with each decade they seemed more and more alien. Yet most Americans saw no need to either accept or reject immigration as such. The problem had not yet been formulated in terms so absolute. Most

16 Jews were active in the intellectual and political revolutions which convulsed Europe at this time, events which conservative Americans also regarded with some ambivalence. Though the Jews fought in a good cause, for freedom of mind and body, "these children of Abraham are for the most part Socialists and infidels—hating Christ with the habitual malignity of the Jew, and the fierce fury of the Jacobin." "Ezra," *Christian Advocate* (New York), April 26, 1849.

17 "Present Influence of the Jews," *Puritan Recorder* (Boston), June 14, 1849.

Americans were still able to maintain a serviceable ambivalence toward immigration and the new citizens that it brought to this country. Americans still had faith in their country and in its God-given mission. No matter how unpromising, how distasteful, Irishmen, or Germans, or Jews might be, all would eventually become Americans. Even those alarmed at the danger to American institutions presented by this immense influx of foreigners still wished to think of their country as a "refuge from European poverty, bigotry or despotism."[18] It was only right that those oppressed in foreign lands "should have better hopes for their children in this country." Providence had chosen this nation to carry out a glorious and peculiar mission. America was to be

an asylum for the oppressed from various parts of the earth—that they might meet here together, blend in one, combine their energies, and establish a more glorious system of society and government than the world ever saw, and throw back their rays of light and influence on the nations whence they sprung.[19]

Disease, most Americans still believed, was but an item in the sum of the immigrants' misfortunes. These foreigners were the victims of dirt and overcrowding, to be pitied not feared. If they were impoverished, it was because Americans allowed them to be exploited. If they died because of their filth and ignorance, it was the duty of Americans to educate and to cleanse them. These unfortunates must be received with charity and understanding, "as Christ commanded and philosophy enjoins." They had fled from man's persecutions to meet in

[18] *Evangelist* (New York), February 1, 1849. Yet less than a month earlier, the same paper had warned that, "this increasing tide of foreigners pouring in upon us is to work changes in our social, moral, and perhaps our political conditions. . . . We are fast losing our identity as Americans, and shall soon fall into a meager and powerless minority. The reins of power and influence are passing from the hands of Americans to those of foreigners" (January 4, 1849).

[19] "The Resources and Destiny of our Country," *Christian Magazine of the South*, VII (1849), 18.

cholera "a more ruthless enemy in a pestilence which preys upon the children of want."[20]

Perhaps the immigrant did find only misery in America's cities. But this was the inevitable result of having never left his port of entry; to remain in the city was to sink ever lower into poverty, crime, and vice. And the nation needed these "stout, strong, and hardy laborers, the very fellows to cut down our forests, cut our railroads, and excavate our canals." While misery increased along the seaboard, "the broad West invites, nay, urges, subsistence and comfort upon the thousands that linger on the spot where they landed."[21] The spot was often the southern tip of Manhattan Island.

It was not surprising that New York suffered from cholera —and typhoid, smallpox, and fevers. "Of all the cities on this continent," wrote a future president of the American Medical Association, "New York stands foremost as the grand focus and receptacle of the poverty and filth of Europe." Disease and civic disorder were the inevitable result. If 1849 had brought cholera and the Astor Place riots, what might succeeding years not bring?[22]

Cities were unnatural and immoral; they bred disease and crime, attracted the vicious, and corrupted the virtuous. These were traditional views, unquestioned by most Americans. Young men were warned of the city's dangers, of evil companions, of drink, and of soul-destroying ambition. Even

[20] Edward H. Dixon, *The Scalpel*, II (1850), 224–25; *Daily Picayune* (New Orleans), January 2, 1849.

[21] *Watchman-Reflector* (Boston), July 5, 1849; *Weekly Herald* (Boston), September 1, 1849.

[22] The symptomatic nature of the Astor Place riots was not lost on conservatives. New York "abounds with the material for mobs and riots," commented a Boston clergyman. "A large proportion of the population is not homogenous—it comprises many men of all nations, and a very great number deplorably ignorant and consequently vicious." *Olive Branch* (Boston), May 19, 1849. Many of the Americans who were alarmed at the dangers of cities took, at the same time, a natural pride in the size and wealth of their cities.

greater were the temptations faced by young women. Jefferson was very much a man of his time in his discomfiture at the moral perils of great cities. The dangers of urban life, so clear in 1800, seemed even more apparent a half-century later.

To such traditional anxiety for the souls of city dwellers had been added a new concern for their bodies. Medical science, with its new statistical tools, had demonstrated irrefutably that the dirt, the congestion, and the bad air of cities shortened men's lives. In England, physicians and social reformers such as Edwin Chadwick, William Farr, and John Simon had made their countrymen conscious of the dangers of poor drainage, foul water, and crowded tenements. Their work and the unashamed empiricism upon which their conclusions were based had, by 1849, helped convince many physicians of the futility of traditional remedies.[23] Disease could not be cured: it must—and could—be prevented through cleanliness and sanitation.

Such teachings seemed increasingly relevant to Americans; their nation was no longer one of farms and villages. America's newer slums already rivaled in filth their European counterparts—even London's notorious tenements harbored no pigs. American city dwellers now seemed less vigorous than their supposedly effete European counterparts. "There is something radically wrong," wrote an Indiana minister, "in the construction of our cities and villages."

The Creator never designed that man should be deprived of the air, and light of heaven. Imperfect ventilation, impure water, and a crowded population, necessarily induce fevers and pestilence; while evil pleasures and sensual pleasures corrupt the morals, and enfeeble the intellect; and generation after generation, fall victims to flagrant violations of the laws of health.[24]

[23] For a useful, brief introduction to the historical development of statistical analysis in medicine and public health, see George Rosen, "Problems in the Application of Statistical Analysis to Questions of Health: 1700–1880," *Bulletin of the History of Medicine*, XXIX (1955), 27–45.

[24] Joseph G. Wilson, *The Voice of God in the Storm, A Discourse Delivered in the Presbyterian Church, on the Day of the National Fast, August 3, 1849* (Lafayette, Ind., 1849), p. 13.

Moral and material causes conspired to produce stunted and rachitic children, adult ill-health, and early death.

An earlier generation had hoped that America might escape such misery. Alexander Stevens, president of the New York State Medical Society, recalled in 1849 his studies in Europe as a young man. It seemed to him then, as he passed through the wards of the London and Paris hospitals, that Americans were hardier and healthier, their climate more salubrious. Thirty-five years later, his opinion had changed: the foul air and filth of American cities and hospitals seemed to have produced the same state of things he had seen as a student in Europe. The continued growth of cities promised, moreover, not only a corresponding increase in bodily ailments, but a disproportionate increase in diseases of the mind.[25] Insanity would, in the city of the future, become as commonplace as malaria in the countryside. (Mental disease was, in the middle of the nineteenth century, frequently attributed to the "artificiality" of urban life.)

Cholera was an extraordinarily lurid sample of the perils that ordinarily menaced the health of tenement dwellers. Twenty Orange Street and the many houses like it merited no particular attention in ordinary times; in the summer of 1849 it was impossible to ignore them, impossible to ignore the connection between the fate of those who died in these tenements and the conditions in which they had lived. Twenty-two pigs made their home in one New York frame building from which five

[25] Stevens, "Annual Address, Delivered before the New-York State Medical Society . . . February 7, 1849," *Transactions of the Medical Society of the State of New York*, 1849, 13–14. The first half of the nineteenth century saw much discussion of whether the growth of civilization increased or decreased disease. Cf., for example, E. H. Ackerknecht, "Hygiene in France, 1815–1848," *Bulletin of the History of Medicine*, XXII (1948), 140–41; Lloyd G. Stevenson, "Science down the Drain," *ibid.*, XXIX (1955), 5–6; Mark D. Altschule, *Roots of Modern Psychiatry* (New York and London, 1957), chap. vii, "The Concept of Civilization as a Social Evil in the Writings of Mid-Nineteenth Century Psychiatrists," pp. 119–39; George Rosen, "Social Stress and Mental Disease from the Eighteenth Century to the Present: Some Origins of Social Psychiatry," *Milbank Memorial Fund Quarterly*, XXXVII (1959), 5–32.

cholera cases were taken. In Philadelphia, "a free couple of color," dying of cholera, were removed from the four and a half by seven foot room in which they lived; in a Boston cellar, the tide rose so high that a physician could only approach a patient's bedside by means of planks laid from one stool to another. The dead body of an infant in its coffin floated in another part of the room.

It was never difficult to predict where, in a city, cholera would first appear. Cholera—and typhoid, smallpox, and typhus—flourished where the ground was low, where garbage was never collected, where there was no adequate ventilation. In Louisville, for example, those sections which suffered most severely in the cholera epidemic of 1833, but which had in the intervening years been cleaned and properly ventilated, suffered not at all in 1849. On the other hand, those squares which were still as dirty as they had been sixteen years before suffered as they had then. Conjectures as to the ultimate cause of cholera were superfluous, and physicians were rebuked for such fruitless disputes "much better calculated to bring ridicule upon the whole profession than to advance the interests of science." Whatever the cause of cholera, it was operative only in close and filthy locations. Epidemics were not inevitable; a perfect system of drainage and sewerage would, reported the secretary of the New Orleans Board of Health, "at once remove all the known causes of disease."[26] It would be cheap at any price.

Millions for defense was a national boast. Yet, charged a committee of the New York State legislature, Americans "grudge the cost of protection against a destroyer more fearful than any mortal foe." Sanitary reform, moreover, had proven its effectiveness. The laws of nature, though immutable, were "beautifully adopted to the welfare of man-

[26] T. S. Bell, "Brief Notes on Cholera in Louisville in 1850," *Western Journal of Medicine*, VI (1850), 104; E. H. Barton, "Annual Report of the New Orleans Board of Health," *Southern Medical Reports*, I (1849), 91.

kind."[27] They had only to be obeyed. So long as city dwellers
allowed filthy tenements and cold, hungry, unwashed people
to exist in their midst, so long would they be scourged by
pestilence. "How the lamp of life, under such circumstances,
holds out to burn, even for a day, is, perhaps, as great a wonder
as that such a state of things should . . . be suffered to exist."[28]
Civilized man could embark upon no task nobler than that of
sanitary reform.[29]

Science had demonstrated that the most malignant epidemics
could be prevented, and it was the responsibility of the legal
guardians of public health to see that they were prevented.
Streets had to be cleaned, cesspools purified, pure water supplied. But no problem was more immediate than that of improving the housing conditions of the poor. Bishop Purcell of
Cincinnati suggested leveling "the filthy and disgusting hovels
where the poor are compelled to congregate, and where, disease is generated and whence it radiates to infect the surrounding atmosphere." These, the Bishop concluded, should be replaced by "whole streets of comfortable cottages." The
Rochester Board of Health suggested the passage of an ordinance requiring all persons wishing to erect a dwelling place to
submit the plans to some competent authority for approval.[30]
Only by improving the living conditions of the poor, it

27 New York State Senate, *Report of the Majority of the Committee on
Medical Societies and Colleges on So Much of the Governor's Message as
Relates to the Cholera* . . . , Doc. No. 92 (Albany, 1850), p. 3; Boston Board
of Health, *op. cit.*, p. 176.

28 Boston Board of Health, *op. cit.*, p. 15.

29 The influential New York *Independent* (November 29, 1849), for example, warned, that "the great practical lesson which the city should have
learned from the cholera," was that ". . . an efficient sanitary police should
be provided which would see to the sanitary condition of the poor, their
tenements and their general physical condition. . . . This is demanded of us
alike by the dictates of humanity and self-interest."

30 Pastoral Letter to the Clergy and Laity of the Diocese of Cincinnati,
July 2, 1849, *Catholic Telegraph*, July 5, 1849; Rochester Board of Health,
Report . . . on Cholera, as It Appeared in Rochester . . . (Rochester, N.Y.,
1852), p. 41.

seemed, could the community protect itself permanently against epidemic disease.

It was clear that the city poor did not live as Americans should. Perhaps, a few Americans suggested, cholera was a judgment demonstrating not that the poor were sinful, but that they were oppressed. That the disease fell most heavily upon the destitute, the intemperate, and the degraded showed not, said Professor Samuel Henry Dickson of New York University, that it was a punishment for sin, but rather that it was "a scourge of our vicious social state."[31] It was "just retribution," wrote the New York *Herald* (July 27, 1849), when cholera spread from "the huts of poverty" to the "palaces of the rich." To reformers, cholera preached a message of social reconstruction; men thought to stop the ravages of cholera

with pestles and mortars, when in deed and in truth the only effectual barricades of resistance were the statute books of nations made comfortable to the statute books of Infinite Justice. It is in a nation's dens of poverty, where unrequited toil pines for its daily food, where nakedness shivers in the wintry air, where the miserable victims of an unjust condition of society hive together in damp cellars and unhealthy garrets, where the blessed air of Heaven is tainted by unventilated streets and dark and obscure lanes and alleys, where pure water is a luxury which the rich only can enjoy, that the cholera is engendered. . . . The great axe of *reform* must be laid at the root of the tree, and this is the lesson which we are to learn from the terrible experiences with which humanity now suffers.[32]

If all men were Christians there would be no cholera: many of those unfortunates dying of cholera were direct sacrifices to Mammon. Criticism of the materialism and amorality of mere wealth was traditional. The remedies offered by accepted wisdom were, however, equally traditional. God must bless the

[31] Samuel H. Dickson, "On the Progress of the Asiatic Cholera during the Years 1844–45–46–47–48," *New York Journal of Medicine,* II (January, 1849), 19.

[32] Thomas Drew, "Our Fast Day Sermon," *Burritt's Christian Citizen* (Worcester, Mass.), August 11, 1849.

rich with honest and liberal hearts and the poor with patience and charity.

Fortunately, however, lives could be saved without disarranging society. Cleanliness, drainage, ventilation, and pure water were goals that could be endorsed by the most moderate. Not only physicians, but every well-informed citizen had been made conscious of the need for improving the conditions of urban life.

Souls as well as bodies would benefit, for physical and spiritual purity were one. Vice was filthy and cleanliness truly next to godliness; the famed piety of the Puritans and Quakers was equaled only by their deserved reputation for cleanliness.

All testimonies agree in affirming that there is scarcely anything more distinctive of paganism than its love of dirt. Catholicism which is but one remove from paganism, shows much of this disgusting character, whether its votaries sun themselves in the streets of Naples, or crouch on the mud floor of an Irish cabin.[33]

"When the Divine Lawgiver communicated with his people by direct revelation," he had been careful to provide them with a complete sanitary code. The recommendations of sanitary commissions and boards of health invariably emphasized the moral benefits that would accrue from improved drains and cesspools. "Bad sanitary regulations," it could not be doubted, had "a certain tendency to degrade the finer moral feelings, and debase individuals towards the level of brute creation."[34]

[33] *Central Watchman* (Cincinnati), July 16, 1849. *Hall's Journal of Health* II (1855), 53–54, warned its readers, for example, never to give charity "*to any dirty person; . . .* deserving poverty is not dirty; if but a rag to wear, there is a mark of care about that rag."

[34] *Western Lancet*, XII (1851), 173. Even so moralistic an improver of the condition of the poor as Robert Hartley, pioneer in urban social welfare organization, never questioned the existence of a connection between physical misery and moral delinquency. "*Social demoralization and crime,* as well as disease, originate and thrive amidst the festering corruptions and pollutions of the miserable accommodations afforded the poor. There is something so congenial in their nature, that 'dirt, disease and crime are concurrent.'" New York Association for Improving the Condition of the Poor, *Eleventh Annual Report . . . for the Year 1854 . . .* (New York, 1854), p. 30.

Perhaps immorality was a product of poverty, of human circumstances rather than human nature. If so, the poor needed medicines, and pure air, and wholesome food before their spiritual regeneration could be attempted. By the same token, prayer and pious injunctions could not alone prevent cholera. Equally futile were the healthful diets, the warm flannels, the scrupulous cleanliness which physicians urged upon the poor; it was a mockery to recommend port, beef roasts, and clean woolens to people sleeping a dozen to a room and eating the refuse of the market places. "Be ye warmed, and be ye clothed," the poor were commanded. Or so it seemed to a growing number of Americans.

Changes in etiological theory also helped to undermine traditional acceptance of personal immorality as a cause of illness. A growing belief in the specificity—though not necessarily the communicability—of disease decreased the physician's reliance upon vague moral factors in explaining its etiology. If the poor suffered most severely from cholera, it was because they were most likely to be exposed to the specific poison. No one would contend that the Five Points had improved either in cleanliness or morality during the years between 1834 and 1849—yet there had been no cholera during these fifteen years despite rum, vice, overflowing cesspools, and manure heaps. Only when a specific material cause was present could cholera appear.[35] At least one rural physician noted that in small towns, where there were no crowded tenements to attract the disease, it was from the ranks of the better and "middling-sort" that cholera chose its victims.[36]

The city's dangers were not inescapable; the miserable and starving tenement dwellers had only to leave for the country

[35] Alexander F. Vache, *Letters on Yellow Fever, Cholera and Quarantine* . . . (New York, 1852), p. 61; New York State Senate, *op. cit.*, p. 30. It will be recalled that few physicians during the 1832 epidemic believed in the existence of particular disease entities.

[36] Joseph C. Hutchinson, "Report on Malignant Cholera, as It Prevailed in Saline County, Mo.," *St. Louis Medical and Surgical Journal*, XI (November, 1853), 489.

to improve at once their own lot and the condition of the city they left. In the West, moreover, the labor of men idle and starving in city slums was desperately needed. It seemed odd that any at all of the laboring poor should remain in the city when the country promised the "certainty (almost) of health and competency." To till the soil was to be one of "nature's real noblemen," to fill "the positon of *a man* in the social structure."[37] The moral advantages of a rural life were as undeniable as its economic ones. Americans were still concerned with individual and moral solutions to social problems. To flee the evils of the city was to solve them.

Few Americans in 1849 questioned the belief that "as a very general rule when a man gets sick it is his own fault, the result of either ignorance or presumption." Immunity from disease lay ultimately in personal habits.[38] Though convinced of the necessity for environmental reform, most thoughtful persons were unable to discard an accustomed belief in the role of moral failing in the causation of disease. To many Americans, for example, it was the slum dweller who was responsible for the filth in which he lived; landlords in more than one city were urged as a preventive of cholera to be more selective in their choice of tenants.

Men's faults were still a possible cause of cholera. Poverty was still, in the eyes of most Americans, a result—not a cause—of vice and imprudence. Cholera was still a judgment.

[37] *American Model Courier* (Philadelphia), June 30, 1849; Joseph G. Wilson, *op. cit.*, p. 17; *Recorder* (Boston), April 6, 1849.

[38] *Hall's Journal of Health*, I (1854), 60. Dr. E. H. Barton, of the New Orleans Board of Health, cited earlier for his belief in the importance of sewerage and drainage improvement, wrote in the same article that every individual carries his safety in his personal habits. "The liability being individual, the municipal power can only aid by cleanliness and ventilation." *Op. cit.*, I, 83.

IX. THE MEDICAL PROFESSION II

Seventeen years pass quickly—even in one man's lifetime. Many American physicians who had survived their first encounter with cholera in 1832, were still practicing in 1849, when the disease next visited the United States. Their tools were of little more use than they had been a generation earlier; their status was lower. But their ideas, even their habits of thought, had begun to change.

The physician had only one assurance in treating cholera: by recognizing and arresting its "premonitory" symptoms, the disease could be anticipated and cured.[1] Were these symptoms ignored, however, and the disease allowed to develop, all remedies would prove useless. Within a few hours after the appearance of the first symptoms, the patient had frequently sunk into collapse—lying prostrate, ashen-faced, and deathly cold. Though they seemed beyond human help, something had to be done for such unfortunates. Many physcians still bled them; a Philadelphia practitioner, for example, when attacked with cholera in the summer of 1849, proceeded to draw sixteen ounces of blood from his own arm. He followed this with a dose of castor oil and the inevitable calomel.[2]

[1] It was "the best, soundest, and most conservative as well as consolatory truth that has hitherto been established relative to spasmodic cholera." Charles Meigs, *Remarks on Spasmodic Cholera* (Philadelphia, 1849), p. 12; Meigs, *Transactions of the College of Physicians of Philadelphia*, II (1849), 433.

[2] George Hamilton, remarks at a meeting of the Philadelphia County Medical Society, October 25, 1865, *Medical and Surgical Reporter*, XIV (1866), 208. Cf. J. Asbury Smith, *American Medical Gazette*, VI (1855), 203.

Calomel was still the "sheet anchor" in the treatment of cholera. Few physicians could do without it; to doughty old Charles Caldwell, removing it from the materia medica would be as disastrous to therapeutics as striking iron from the list of metals would be to mechanics.[3] Nevertheless, calomel was rarely prescribed alone, but usually in conjunction with laudanum, cayenne pepper, or jalap—remedies equally unpleasant.

Many physicians disdained such trite practice. They seized upon the novel, upon anything which promised to cure. And an American, a Chicagoan, contributed what seemed to be the most promising of such remedies—sulphur. A determinedly scientific explanation by its discoverer, a Dr. Byrd, had proven —to Dr. Byrd's satisfaction—that a deficiency of ozone in the atmosphere caused cholera; only sulphur, he believed, could counteract this pernicious condition. Within a month of the publication of this discovery, sulphur pills, even sulphur candies, could be purchased from Maine to Texas.[4] Unfortunately, this comparatively harmless enthusiasm was scorned by the more imaginative among the medical fraternity. One Alabama practitioner relied upon tobacco-smoke enemas, an Ohio physician upon electric shocks, while others swore by strychnine, or aconite, or morphine. Even more extreme were the doctors who immersed their comatose patients in tubs of ice water.[5]

But protests were increasing. Even within the medical profession, critical minds were beginning to question the utility of traditional remedies—especially bleeding and calomel. When we knew a little of cholera, a skeptical physician remarked, we prescribed a few grains of calomel "now and then." Now that time had proven we knew even less of the

3 Caldwell, *Autobiography* . . . (Philadelphia, 1855), p. 184.

4 The original article appeared in the *Chicago Journal*, May 29, 1849.

5 For a few of these extreme forms of treatment, see, H. L. Byrd, "The Therapeutical Application of Electro-Magnetism in Cholera," *Charleston Medical Journal*, VIII (1853), 628–30; Charles J. Hempel, *Tribune* (New York), June 7, 1849; *North-Western Journal of Homoeopathy*, I (1849), 202 f.; John L. Page, *Buffalo Medical and Surgical Journal*, V (1866), 207–8; John W. Moore, *Alabama Planter* (Mobile), January 8, 1849.

disease, he concluded, patients were given teaspoonfuls.[6] Many physicians conceded that they could do little for those stricken with cholera. Claims of extraordinary cures, they charged, were due either to wilful misrepresentation or to their author's unfamiliarity with real Asiatic cholera. The director of one of New York's cholera hospitals came to rely upon beef tea— and the *vis medicatrix naturae*. "If the patient have not the constitution to resist the attack, we can't create it: if his system will not react, therapeutics must be powerless in his case."[7] Patients died at the same rate regardless of the therapy employed. Hospital statistics had demonstrated conclusively this sad truth.

Statistics were becoming the reality of science. Their use within the medical profession at once expressed and justified an increasingly critical temper; accepted theories and remedies must be proven effective—and if not, discarded. The spirit as well as the achievements of the great Paris clinicians, especially Pierre Louis and his "numerical" method, had inspired their American disciples. Such questioning minds were horrified at the quality, rather than reassured by the quantity, of American medical effusions on cholera.

We find often no statistics of numbers, ages, sexes, colours, no numerical ratio of attacks to recoveries, no proofs of the value of remedies, beyond assertions and boastings, no autopsies, no tracking of an epidemic from the first cases to its probable cause, no report of the sequence of cases, where in a very limited locality, the knowledge might be very easily obtained. . . .[8]

[6] Edward Dixon, *The Scalpel*, II (1850), 251.

[7] Joseph C. Hutchinson, "History and Observations on Asiatic Cholera in Brooklyn . . . ," *New York Journal of Medicine*, XIV (1855), 70.

[8] Committee on Practical Medicine, *Transactions of the American Medical Association*, III (1850), 107. Cf. John K. Mitchell, *Introductory Lecture Delivered in Jefferson Medical College of Philadelphia, October 16, 1849* (Philadelphia, 1849), p. 17. For an evaluation of the impact of the Paris clinical school on American medicine, see Richard H. Shryock, *Medicine and Society in America 1660–1860* (New York, 1960), pp. 123 ff. Louis, it should be noted, was a particular favorite with American students.

Unfortunately for the medical profession, few physicians allowed such skepticism to affect their practice. "Therapeutic nihilism," the doctrinaire disbelief in the efficacy of traditional remedies, was limited to the intellectually ruthless in academic medicine; it held few attractions for the average practitioner, who had necessarily to do something for his patients. Even those willing to acknowledge that medicines were probably of little use continued to prescribe them—and won few friends among the public.[9]

Never before had the status of the American medical profession been as low.[10] In 1832, few well-educated and respectable Americans would have consulted any but a regularly educated physician. Less than two decades later, hydropathic and homeopathic physicians were welcome in some of the most respectable American homes. The most obvious cause of this deterioration in its standing was the imperfections of the medical profession itself. But these had not changed greatly in the twenty years between 1830 and 1850; other less obvious causes must be sought within a rapidly changing American society.

None were more conscious of their declining status than the doctors themselves. But a few short years before, lamented a mid-century Ohio physician, there had been something dignified and reassuring in the word "physician." Now, like the porter, his services were calculated by the hour and grudgingly rewarded. The "stately step, the solemn look, the 'big gold-headed cane,' and 'consequential air'" were no longer sufficient to command respect in the public mind.[11] With the excep-

[9] For an excellent survey of changes in therapeutic practice, see Alex Berman, "The Heroic Approach in 19th Century Therapeutics," *Bulletin of the American Society of Hospital Pharmacists*, September–October, 1954, 321-27.

[10] This is a fact well known to the historian. Not so well known is the rapidity of the decline that it underwent in the years between 1830 and 1850. See, for example, the discussion by Richard H. Shryock, in "Public Relations of the Medical Profession in Great Britain and the United States: 1600-1870," *Annals of Medical History*, II (1930), 308-39; and Shryock, *The Development of Modern Medicine* (New York, 1947), chap. xiii, "Public Confidence Lost."

[11] John Dawson, *Western Journal of Medicine*, III (1849), 486.

tion of those few practitioners whose personal dignity or professional attainments disarmed criticism, most physicians were
regarded as ill-educated and unethical quacks.

Doctors, like lawyers, had always served as a target for the
resentment and humor of the cynical. But never, it seemed, had
public unanimity and bitterness been as great. Physicians were,
in the words of one popular saying, the nutcrackers used by
angels to get our souls out of the shells surrounding them.
Cholera was a most terrible affliction, commented James Gordon Bennett's *Herald* (August 12, 1849), but bad doctors and
bad drugs were worse. The pestilence might come now and
then; physicians we had always with us. Unfortunately for the
medical profession, such sentiments inspired more than irreverent repartee.

South Carolina and Maryland in 1838 and New York in
1844 removed all legal restrictions upon the practice of medicine. By 1851, fifteen states in all had repealed such regulatory
legislation; eight others had never passed any. When, in 1851,
the Georgia legislature appropriated $5,000 for a Botanic
Medical College, the nadir seemed to have been reached.[12] And
the protests of regular physicians had a self-serving ring.

Even the most credulous of Americans had become skeptical of the physicians' claims to the dignity of a learned profession. The requirements for graduation from medical school,
complained a Massachusetts physician, were purely nominal,
the final examination a "mere pretense." In Iowa, six months of
reading medicine were sufficient to win the title of doctor. The
prospective healer then bought a "pound of calomel, an ounce
of quinine, a drachm of morphine," and considered himself
ready to locate. It is acknowledged on all hands, remarked a
Memphis physician, "that we are a *rapid*, not to say fast people.
. . . We are *rapid* in dollars and cents; rapid on land and on sea;

[12] *Western Journal of Medicine*, X (1852), 183; Richard H. Shryock, "Public Relations of the Medical Profession . . . ," *Annals of Medical History*, N.S.
II, 322; Donald E. Konold, "A History of American Medical Ethics 1847–
1912" (unpublished doctoral dissertation, University of Missouri, 1954), pp.
24–25.

rapid in eating and drinking, and thinking; but our rapidity in making doctors is above all things wonderful."[13] The requirements for entrance into even the leading medical schools were at best rudimentary; the aspiring medical student was often unread, sometimes almost illiterate.[14] After graduation, the average physician rarely subscribed to medical journals and infrequently purchased books, relying on those texts he had acquired in his student days.

It was not only knowledge the ordinary physician lacked. His dignity, bearing, and ethics often reflected scant credit on either himself or his profession. One's local practitioner might, in the words of a disillusioned colleague, "be uncouth in his manners, vulgar and indelicate in his language, slovenly in his dress, and harsh and unfeeling in his treatment."[15] Wealthy patients were eagerly pursued, while many physicians refused to make night calls or to treat the poor. Others paid for adulatory items in local newspapers or sold secret remedies—practices denounced as marks of quackery in those outside the regular profession. In cholera times especially, the doctors were convenient targets for public fear and frustration. Some fled. The greater number of physicians remained faithful, however, only to be criticized for manufacturing cholera cases in order to increase their reputation—or for concealing cases to the same end. Almost all physicians were criticized for their harsh remedies.

More damaging to the medical profession than either lack of education or of ethical standards was the practice of the average physician. His ministrations provided neither cure nor the

13 *Memphis Medical Recorder*, II (1853), 137; I. F. Galloupe, "One Cause of Empiricism," *Boston Medical and Surgical Journal*, XLI (December 12, 1849), 379–82.

14 The Baltimore *Sun*, July 28, 1849 printed some of the more egregious errors in spelling and syntax from New York City cholera reports. Editors of medical journals complained constantly of the ignorance and apathy of the average physician. For a survey of American medical education in this period, see William T. Norwood, *Medical Education in the United States before the Civil War* (Philadelphia, 1944).

15 Dan King, *Boston Medical and Surgical Journal*, XL (June 13, 1849), 370.

illusion of competence and consistency: five different physicians attending the same case would, according to popular belief, invariably present the helpless patient with five different prescriptions—alike only in their unpleasantness. Calomel was so unpopular that physicians were forced to devise artful strategems to induce their patients to take it.[16] And the doses were immense; a common rule of thumb warned that the drug had not begun to take effect until the patient's gums bled.

Its lack of dignity and of education, even its harsh remedies, could have been forgiven the medical profession had it produced results. But its failures were too conspicuous. Skeptical Americans found little to justify the exclusive pretensions of a profession unable to provide even the assurance of unanimity; medicine seemed the least exact and most backward of the sciences. Surgery, not surprisingly, with its standardized procedures and often verifiable results, was exempt from much of the criticism accorded the practice of medicine. One New Yorker, for instance, who had nothing but contempt for most physicians, professed a real admiration for the surgeon. For, he argued,

if a limb be dislocated or shattered, an artery punctured, or a bullet 'propelled' into a gentleman's midriff, we know that the surgeon, with his splints and bandages, his tourniquet, or his probe and knife, as the case may be, is not only a useful, but an absolutely necessary agent.

Moreover, he continued significantly, "there is but one method of setting a limb, of taking up an artery, or of extracting a bullet; and upon this method all well-educated surgeons are agreed."[17]

Not that ordinary folk lacked faith in drugs. Many, for example, believed that physicians took some mysterious potion which protected them during epidemics. It was impossible to

---

[16] Even eminent physicians found it difficult to secure patients if they were reputed to prescribe large doses of calomel. *Hall's Journal of Health*, I (1854), 208.

[17] *Sunday Times* (New York), December 31, 1848.

wean the "common people" from their traditional belief in the necessary existence of a specific remedy for every disease. And it was to this belief that the patent-medicine vender appealed. In the vocabulary of the regular practitioner, "specific," "empiric," and "quack" were roughly synonymous. "The search for a *specific for cholera in all its stages* would be as vain as that of the ancient alchemists for the philosopher's stone, or any of the visionary enterprises of the knight of La Mancha. It is a *humbug* resorted to alone by designing charlatans who would batten on the ignorance and credulity of the people."[18] The educated physician scorned specifics, treating disease through general physiological principles—principles unknown to the untutored empiric. Unfortunately, these principles were equally mysterious to a public unable to understand how five different remedies might legitimately be employed in treating the same patient if all served the same purpose—the reduction of fever, let us say. Such medical reasoning and the education it implied had helped undershore the status of the physician in earlier centuries. But it produced no results and seemed no more than self-serving obscurantism to many Americans in 1849.

There had always been a market for secret remedies. But it was not until the 1840's that the sale of individual patent medicines became nationwide. America's cheap and ubiquitous newspapers had made this possible. In more primitive times, such remedies rarely attained a more than local reputation; advertising, too, was local. By mid-century, the patent-medicine entrepreneurs had become the first of the national advertisers. The reassuring whiskers of Old Jacob Townsend—not to mention his sarsaparilla—were as well known in Texas and Iowa as

[18] Thomas Sydenham's search for specific remedies was, at this time, considered his major failing, though the reputation of this great English clinician was otherwise unimpeached. Knud Faber, *Nosography* (2d ed. rev.; New York, 1930), p. 109. "Paracelsus" was, as might have been expected, another synonym for quack. Respectable physicians justified their categorical rejection of specific remedies by maintaining that the age and sex of the patient, the climate and season, the stage of the disease, had all to be taken into account in deciding the nature and dosage of medicines.

in New York.[19] Such advertising was one of the few reliable sources of income for most newspaper editors—a substitution for the government printing denied those unfortunates who had backed the wrong party. Grateful editors filled their columns with puffs for purges and tonics and jibes at the regular medical profession.

The doctors were not to be trusted. There was only one solution, editors warned—every American must study the laws of health and disease for himself. And none outside the regular medical profession was more zealous in such self-improvement than the clergy. Not only did they continue, in some cases, to do a bit of their own doctoring, as clergymen had for centuries, they endorsed patent medicines and supported heterodox medical systems. Far less influential than the clergy in mid-nineteenth-century America, the medical profession could do little in retaliation.[20]

But the clergy were not alone in having withdrawn support from the medical profession. Seventeen years before, in 1832, Thomsonian or botanic medicine was the only unorthodox medical system with any real following in this country. Though popular, botanic medicine had been a rural and lower-class phenomenon, an enthusiasm of the vulgar and almost destitute of respectable support. By 1850, however, hydropathic and homeopathic physicians could boast of substantial follow-

[19] The most recent and extensive survey of the patent-medicine business is that by James Harvey Young, *The Toadstool Millionaires: A social history of patent medicines in America before federal regulation* (Princeton, 1961).

[20] Though he complained of declining prestige as well, the minister was still far more influential, as a rule, than the physician, who labored under the traditional stigma of materialism and infidelity. See, for example, "Curio," *Whig* (Richmond), July 18, 1849; Thomas Steel to James Steel, January 21, 1849, Thomas Steel Papers, Manuscript Division, State Historical Society of Wisconsin; J. H. Stuart, "Cholera Asphyxia," *New Jersey Medical Reporter*, VI (1853), 114; J. S. Sprague, "Annual Address," *Transactions of the Medical Society of the State of New York*, 1854, p. 12. More symptomatic than effectual were the frequent threats made by local medical societies to discontinue their traditionally gratuitous treatment of clergymen who endorsed patent medicines or supported sectarian rivals.

ings among the well to do, a claim tacitly endorsed by the imprecations of the regular faculty.[21]

How can so rapid a change be explained? The most apparent cause was the imperfect state of the medical profession itself. Pragmatic Americans could scarcely fail to note that their average physician was neither healer nor scholar.

But in this he had not changed greatly in the years since 1832. It was America that had changed. Traditional class distinctions had been weakened: the equalitarian and centrifugal tendencies of Jacksonian America had not only undercut the standards of the medical profession, but had eroded as well the conservative convictions of an earlier generation. Successful Americans no longer assumed without question the desirability of a stable graded society. No longer did maintaining the status of the learned professions play a part—a necessary part—in maintaining the stability of society itself.

Most Americans had come to accept without question the virtues of progress and equalitarianism; and these values seemed to deny the "exclusive pretensions" of the regular physicians. In the rhetoric of their "sectarian" competitors, the medical profession was identified with blind conservatism and opposition to change. Medical schismatics pictured themselves as victims of intolerance and obscurantism, the Galileos and Giordano Brunos of a supposedly enlightened nineteenth century. Now, however, charged one dissident, the worst that the regulars could do was to slander us. "Time was," he continued, "when we should have been kindly caged in cold, damp, cells with bread and water for our diet; or had our limbs amiably broken on a wheel, or have been benevolently burnt at the stake."[22] Traditional medical science was an "antiquated

21 A petition to the New York City Board of Health appealing for the establishment of a hospital on homeopathic principles during the 1849 cholera epidemic was signed by such prominent New Yorkers as W. C. Bryant, P. J. Van Rensselaer, Stephen Cambreleng, and General James Talmadge—all trustees of the Homoeopathic Dispensary Association. File Drawer U-60, City Clerk's Papers, Municipal Archives and Records Center, contains the original petitions, dated June 8 and June 14.

22 William Turner, *Revelations on Cholera* . . . , ed. Samuel Dickson (New York, 1849), p. 61.

heathen humbug, utterly unworthy of the middle of the nine-teenth century."[23]

Doctorcraft, like priestcraft would have to be swept away. "We go in for the 'largest liberty,' " affirmed a Cincinnati jour-nalist, "without pretending to decide which system is the best." Liberals everywhere, he continued, "desire that medicine, like theology, should be divorced from State, and that, as in the different sects of religionists, the various medical systems shall be treated alike. . . . We go for free trade in doctoring." It was encouraging to critics of a seemingly authoritarian medical profession to see state after state abolishing "discriminatory" medical legislation; to repeal such restrictive enactments was to leave "reason and public opinion as the sole legislators of the medical profession."[24]

Homeopathy, the most widespread of the medical sects competing with the regular profession, benefited as well from a rapidly increasing German immigration, which provided both patients and practitioners. Like hydropathy, moreover, homeopathy was comparatively inexpensive and at worst harm-less. At least homeopathic medicines would "not make well men sick, nor keep sick men from getting well."[25] The same could hardly be said of traditional remedies.

Hydropathy, though like homeopathy of European origin,

[23] *Sunday Dispatch* (New York), January 7, 1849.

[24] *Daily Times* (Cincinnati), n.d., cited in the *Physiologico-Medical Re-corder*, XVII (1849), 175–76, 196. Though most Americans were hostile to the medical profession, such extreme Jacksonian-enlightenment rhetoric can be found only in those publications which consciously appealed to the "com-mon people."

[25] *Christian Ambassador*, II (1849), 443; *Olive Branch* (Boston), March 31, 1849; *Wisconsin Free Democrat* (Milwaukee), December 13, 1848. Homeop-athy, which still survives in an attenuated form, was a medical system founded late in the eighteenth century by Samuel Hahnemann, a German physician. Its therapy was based upon the assumption that diseases could be cured by drugs that caused in the well person symptoms similar to those of the dis-ease. More important practically was Hahnemann's conviction that the strength of a drug increased with dilution. (The influence of Jenner and vaccination for smallpox upon this doctrine seems likely.) It was clear to even the bitterest enemies of homeopathy that its medicines were harmless. The same had to be admitted of the baths and diets of the hydropaths.

appealed most strongly to the spiritually committed, the reformers and moral absolutists—"ultras" in contemporary slang. Abolition in politics and pure water in medicine were frequently found together, for their advocates saw them as moral, not political or scientific, issues. Truth, affirmed the editor of the *Water-Cure Journal* was always "ultra."[26] God's pure and wholesome water was as superior to "filthy," "unnatural," and dangerous drugs as it was to whiskey, or as freedom was to slavery. It is no accident that both abolitionism and medical sectarianism first gained wide public acceptance in the years between 1832 and 1850. This was an earnest generation: the millennial zeal of an earlier day had faded, but not without leaving behind many Americans unable to compromise with sin, immorality, or imperfection in any form. The orthodox in medicine, in religion, and in politics were alike impeding the attainment of God's kingdom on earth.[27]

[26] R. T. Trall, *Water-Cure Journal*, VII (1849), 88. The *Wisconsin Free Democrat* (Milwaukee), the *Model Worker* (Utica, N.Y.), *National Era* (Washington, D.C.), *Non-Resistant* (Milford, Mass.), *Burritt's Christian Citizen*, and the *Evangelist* and *Independent* (New York) were some of the "reforming" publications which supported hydropathy. See, also, Thomas H. Le Duc, "Grahamites and Garrisonites," *New York History*, XX (1939), 189–91; and Alex Berman, "Social Roots of the 19th Century Botanico-medical Movement in the United States," *Actes du VIIIᵉ Congrés International d'Histoire des Sciences*, September 1956, pp. 561–65. Their sectarian opponents called the members of the regular medical profession "hunkers"—the same name given the anti-free-soil wing of New York's Democratic party by political antagonists.

[27] One sort of *"ism* generally begets another," commented a physician orthodox in religion as well as in medicine. S. W. Butler, "Organized Quackery.—How should it be dealt with?" *New Jersey Medical Reporter*, VI (1853), 105–6. See, also, Alonzo S. Ball, *The Present Position of the Two Schools of Medicine* . . . (Albany, 1854), pp. 24–25. The connection between orthodoxy in medicine and orthodoxy in religion was clear to contemporaries. See, for example, Charles Anderson to Caleb B. Smith, July 3, 1849, Caleb B. Smith Papers, Library of Congress. Or, as one abolitionist commented, ". . . We would as soon trust our spirit to a regular parson as our body to a pill-peddler. There are honest men everywhere, of course. But they are hard to find, in the medical, as well as in the clerical and legal professions." *Model Worker* (Utica, N.Y.), December 8, 1849.

The postmillennial rhetoric of the "ultras" was not, of course, identical with the earlier patterns of Enlightenment rhetoric utilized by the Thomsonians. It is, however, difficult in practice to disentangle the two styles of argument. The earlier Thomsonian writings appealed to a class bias and class

During cholera times, the medical profession's stubborn defense of its prerogatives seemed particularly self-seeking. In a number of cities, public health efforts had been paralyzed by squabbles between the regular and homeopathic physicians; in Milwaukee, Columbus, and Cincinnati, boards of health had to be reconstituted completely. Perhaps accord could be reached only by banning physicians from sitting on such boards; this was no time for ruffled dignity and jealous guarding of prerogative. "The public cares little, whether Dr. Sangrado is pitied by Dr. Bolus, or if Dr. Allopathy sneers at Dr. Homeopathy."[28] "If either allopathy or homeopathy or hydropathy, or any common-sense-pathy will help to secure us . . . in the name of mercy let us have the one pathy that will do it."[29]

More than a few physicians despaired of such a nation.[30] America seemed the natural home of humbug. Many regular practitioners could not help but question the values of a society that justified quackery and denigrated their own faithful efforts. Could one acknowledge as infallible a public opinion which seemed to demand charlatanry as the price of success? Under the guise of "progress," the Goths and Vandals of modern barbarism had succeeded in investing the last strongholds of science.

As we are well aware, these bastions were not to fall. The

---

consciousness in a way that would have been unacceptable to many Americans willing to patronize hydropathy or homeopathy. Though willing to accept the logic of equalitarianism, moderates in mid-century America avoided the class-consciousness that often accompanied it a generation earlier. They emphasized instead the unity and mutual dependency of all classes in society.

[28] [William L. Robinson], *Diary of a Samaritan* (New York, 1860), p. 77. On the break-up of local health boards, see *Ohio State Journal* (Columbus), July 25, 1849; *Weekly Wisconsin* (Milwaukee), July 25, 1849; Peter T. Harstad, "Disease and Sickness on the Wisconsin Frontier: Cholera," *Wisconsin Magazine of History*, XLIII (1960), 203–20; Thomas Carroll, "Cholera as It Appeared in Cincinnati in 1849," *Cincinnati Lancet and Observer*, IX (1866), 298 f.

[29] *Sun* (New York), July 30, 1849.

[30] Most physicians, of course, shared the social preconceptions of their fellow Americans. Their attacks on sectarian rivals thus seemed ambivalent, unconvincing, and ultimately self-serving.

American respect for tangible results which had been so instrumental in destroying public confidence in the medical profession was, within a century, to raise the physician's status to unprecedented heights. But this knowledge would have been at best an ironic consolation to the physician in mid-nineteenth-century America. His was a hostile world, a world turned upside down, in which democracy and morality, reason and progress, the very ideals he lived by, had become the allies of quackery and humbug.

Everyone wrote on cholera. Indeed, the subject seemed almost to have been exhausted. The writer of a treatise on cholera, complained one medical author in 1849, was in much the same position as the prospective author of a Fourth of July oration or a eulogy of General Washington. There was nothing new to say.

But not all American physicians were so discouraged. In the seventeen years since cholera's first appearance in North America, chemistry and biology had provided new alternatives to older ideas.[31] The work of Bassi and Ehrenberg on microorganisms, of Berzelius and Liebig on fermentation and catalysis, was known, even if in popularized form. Advances in clinical medicine and pathology had also begun to exert an important influence, making respectable the idea of disease specificity.[32] (In addition, experience with so striking a disease

31 On the whole, however, the etiological thinking of most American physicians had not changed greatly since 1832. One hundred and three of one hundred and forty-six physicians sampled considered the disease non-contagious. Twenty-three considered it to be primarily contagious, while twenty held that it could become so in some circumstances.

Of the one hundred and forty-six opinions tabulated, thirty-three did not state clearly what they felt to be the cause of the disease. Thirty-five favored some atmospheric influence, while sixteen held a miasma responsible. Seven suggested a deficiency—or an excess—of electricity in the atmosphere. Four physicians considered a lack of oxygen—or an excess of nitrogen—to be the cause of cholera. Five held fungi or animalculi responsible, while three attributed it to "a specific animal poison." Four doctors considered microscopic "germs" to be the cause of the disease.

32 The Americans who had studied in the Paris clinics in the 1830's were the apostles of a critical spirit of scientific inquiry—and the teachers of a new generation of medical students. As has been discussed, however, specificity in

had convinced many during the first cholera pandemic of its
specificity. Cholera was, in the words of Sir Thomas Watson,
a "malady . . . too striking, to be overlooked, or ever forgotten,
by any who had once seen it.")[33] By 1849, most physicians
agreed that cholera was a specific disease caused by a specific
poison.

Still, ideas of specificity were hardly rigid; to many, the
variability of disease remained an article of faith. It was difficult to believe that disease could remain the same, while social,
even geological and climatic, conditions changed. "Constitutions, and habits of life, and modes of living are constantly
changing; hence new diseases are making their appearance
from time to time, while others have vanished from the
world."[34] Many observers still noted that influenza and intestinal disorders heralded cholera's arrival. And, as a physician
warned President Polk, "all diseases of the bowels had a
tendency to run into cholera when that disease prevailed."[35]

The great majority of physicians still believed that the cause
of cholera lay in the atmosphere. But now the mere profession
of this belief seemed inadequate. Believers had to be more precise: they could no longer rely alone on affirmation and intona-
tion, but must attempt to define whatever it was in the atmosphere that caused the disease. The number of physicians content to assign the disease to an "epidemic influence" or an "im-
ponderable atmospheric peculiarity" decreased markedly.

---

therapy still bore the stigma of quackery. For the best short survey of the
advances in clinical medicine associated with the Paris school, see Knud Faber,
Nosography (2d ed. rev.; New York, 1930).

[33] Watson, *Lectures on the Principles and Practice of Physic* (Philadelphia,
1844), p. 718. J. W. Francis, for example, a prominent New York physician,
wrote of cholera in 1832 that "nosology could not classify a more distinctive
disease." *Letters on Cholera* . . . (New York, 1832), p. 32.

[34] *Hall's Journal of Health*, I (1854), 189–90.

[35] Milo M. Quaife (ed.), *The Diary of James K. Polk* . . . (Chicago, 1910),
IV, 412. A Dr. McCall of Nashville expressed a typical attitude when he wrote
that "it certainly has traits *sui generis*, and yet combines with and aggravates
all other maladies present." "Remarks on Asiatic Cholera," *Western Lancet*,
IX (1849), 15.

Now one charged the disease to electricity, or ozone, or carbonic acid, or at least a "specific aeriform poison."[36] Local exciting causes continued, however, to play a prominent role in etiological thinking. To a generation increasingly conscious of the relationship between disease and environment, local filth and lack of ventilation and pure water were the obvious reasons for the concentration of cholera cases in circumscribed slum areas.

But moral as well as physical causes might induce cholera. Journalists and ministers, as well as physicians, published exhaustive catalogues of the disreputable actions that might lead to the disease. Newspaper readers were urged to "have peace with God, through the Lord Jesus Christ," for "your peace will be of essential service in enabling you to throw off the malady." The doctrine of predisposing causes was completely unquestioned by the medical profession. Even the moderate report of the American Medical Association's Committee on Practical Medicine and Epidemics reasoned that cholera could not be contagious, for a debauch or a drinking bout had never been known to cause a *contagious* disease.[37]

Other, older patterns of thought endured as well. There were still few who questioned the assumption that an epidemic disease drove out other diseases or made them "wear its livery." (Epidemics "seem ever to exercise upon the atmosphere a controlling power, as exemplified in the fact that the ordinary diseases of the country partake in some measure, of the character of the prevailing epidemic.")[38] When cholera was

36 Such ideas, of course, clearly reflect the influence of contemporary progress in the natural sciences. In New York City, for example, the Board of Health engaged a professor of chemistry to analyze the atmosphere during the epidemic. New York Board of Health, *Report of the . . . Sanatory Committee . . .* (New York, 1849), pp. 59 f.

37 *Evangelist* (New York), June 14, 1849; *Transactions of the American Medical Association*, III (1850), 127–29.

38 Frank A. Ramsey, *Cholera* (Knoxville, 1849), p. 2. See also W. H. Scoby, "Remarks on the Influence of Cholera on other Diseases," *Western Lancet*, XI (1850), 91–93; John Butterfield, *Ohio Medical and Surgical Journal*, I (1849), 576; A. G. Lawton, "On the Epidemic Cholera," *American Medical Monthly*, III (1855), 182. In the East and in large cities, these ideas

epidemic, a popular saying consoled, all other diseases disappeared. Rather than increasing, the bills of mortality were less crowded than usual.

As had not been the case in 1832, however, a few critics made themselves heard: the Philadelphia Board of Health proved, by a comparison of mortality statistics for the years 1846 through 1849, that cholera had not driven out other diseases, but that they had, on the contrary, increased during the cholera year.[39] Observers in New York and Brooklyn also noted that cholera did not swallow up other diseases or force them to wear its livery. Moreover, fundamental criticisms of the atmospheric theory itself became frequent.

It was only an excuse for thought, said Alexander Stevens, president of the New York State Medical Association in 1849 —and a believer in the atmospheric origin of cholera in 1832. "It is improperly called an explanation," he continued, "it is only a confession of ignorance; and just as strong proof might be adduced that diseases were induced by witchcraft, or the influence of comets and fiery dragons in the heavens; . . . it should be discarded from science; it belongs to the dark ages." John Evans, editor of the *North-Western Medical and Surgical Journal*, charged the atmosphere with having been "made the scape-goat to bear off the sins of our ignorance." What evidence, he asked, had ever been presented for this theory other than the fact that everyone contracts cholera while breathing; one might as well blame the stars or the moon for having caused the disease.[40]

The rhetoric of progress could cut two ways, however, and

were no longer entertained with such assurance. For example, the four physicians cited in this note hail, respectively, from Knoxville, Tennessee, Rossville, Ohio, Columbus, Ohio, and La Salle, Illinois.

[39] Philadelphia Board of Health, *Statistics of Cholera* . . . (Philadelphia, 1849), p. 47. The use of such statistics is, of course, more significant than any particular conclusions which their users may have reached.

[40] Stevens, "On the Communicability of Asiatic Cholera," *Transactions of the Medical Society of New York*, 1850, p. 33; *North-Western Medical and Surgical Journal*, II (1849), 278.

the anticontagionists were the ones who employed it most frequently in their attacks on quarantine regulations. The quarantines implied by a belief in contagionism were regarded with some ambivalence even by contagionists, while their opponents labeled them inhuman "relicts of barbarism and superstition." It seemed indeed a mystery "that this absurd system [was] still maintained, in spite of all sense, science and experience." The abolition of quarantines was a triumph "of truth over error, not only for the honor of the human mind, but for the benefits of commerce; and above all for the good of humanity."[41]

By 1849, the idea that cholera was "portable," though not contagious, seemed a moderate one, consistent with the great bulk of evidence. Even decided anticontagionists had to account for this portability. Especially in rural and isolated communities, the circumstances surrounding cholera outbreaks pointed unmistakably to its having been imported from infected areas.[42]

Nevertheless, there were anomalies in the spread of this "portable" disease not easily explained by believers in either the contagionist or atmospheric theories. Fortunately, the natural sciences had provided new explanations. One, stemming from biology and microscopy, suggested that a micro-organism, either plant or animal, might be responsible for causing the disease. The second, originating in the work of chemists on catalysis and fermentation, conceived of the epidemic as a

[41] The sources of the three quotations are, respectively, *St. Louis Medical and Surgical Journal*, IX (1851), 418; *Bulletin* (New Orleans), July 28, 1849; *Southern Medical Journal*, III (April, 1839), 423. And, as compared with 1832, the enforcement of quarantines was allowed to lapse, as public health efforts were bent toward the attainment of cleanliness and purity. Where quarantines existed in America in 1849, it was usually at the insistence of the vulgar; where enforced at all, it was in an erratic fashion.

[42] For the spread of cholera in rural areas, see George Sutton, "A Report to the Indiana State Medical Society on Asiatic Cholera, as It Prevailed in This State in 1849–50–51–52," *Proceedings of the Indiana State Medical Society*, 1853, p. 115; *New Jersey Chronicle* (Bridgeton), July 21, 1849; D. P. Holloway to Caleb B. Smith, August 4, 1849, Caleb B. Smith Papers, Library of Congress; *People's Friend* (Covington, Ind.), August 25, 1849; *Democratic Expounder* (Marshall, Mich.), August 3, 1849.

kind of delayed chemical reaction, taking place either in the atmosphere or the patient's body and caused by the introduction of a small amount of cholera "ferment" or "catalyst."

The idea that microscopic organisms might cause disease was a novel but not entirely new one to American medical thinkers in 1849. As early as 1836, John L. Riddell, adjunct professor of chemistry at the Cincinnati Medical College, had outlined at some length a theory in which diseases were caused by "corpuscles," "trans-microscopic" in size, which held "nearly the same grade in respect to animate sentient beings which the more simple and minute of the *Fungi* and *Algae* do to the more perfect tribe of vegetables."[43] The cause of cholera must, he reasoned, be organic, for only in living organisms is found the ability to reproduce indefinitely.

In the fall of 1849, readers of the Philadelphia *Medical Examiner* would have come across an editorial marshaling the evidence for the idea that a micro-organism was the cause of cholera. Reference was made to the work of Bassi, Schönlein, and Henle, and even to a German biologist, who had, as early as 1832, found microscopic fungi in the dejecta of cholera patients. The article concluded with a notice of the recent publications of Dr. William Budd; the English physician had, it seemed, adopted the "fungoid theory" and suggested that the spread of cholera could be prevented by placing cholera evacuations in a chemical fluid known to be fatal to the "fungous tribe."[44]

[43] "Memoir on the Nature of Miasm and Contagion," *Western Journal of Medical and Physical Sciences*, IX (1835), 401–12, 526–32. Riddell had obviously been reading the publications of European investigators on infusoria and fermentation. Cf. Phyllis Allen, "Americans and the Germ Theory of Disease" (unpublished doctoral thesis, University of Pennsylvania, 1949); and Allen, "Early American Animalcular Hypotheses," *Bulletin of the History of Medicine*, XXI (1947), 734–43.

[44] *Medical Examiner*, V (1849), 685–88. Dr. Budd also suggested that water should be supplied from uninfected districts, for it was "the principal channel through which this poison finds its way into the human body." Dr. Budd, it will be recalled, was later to gain fame for his studies of the means of transmission of typhoid fever.

Agostino Bassi, an Italian lawyer, had shown in 1835 that fungi caused a disastrous silkworm disease; J. L. Schönlein, a German physician, had proven

The fungous or cryptogamous theory was, in the United States, identified with the name of Dr. John Kearsley Mitchell. A professor at Jefferson Medical College, Mitchell suggested that cholera and other diseases were, in all probability, caused by a fungus, the spores of which could be wafted from place to place through the atmosphere.[45] Other physicians, though willing to assume that the cause of cholera was organic, were not able to accept Mitchell's fungi. Some considered "Infusoria" or "animalcula" the cause, while others were unwilling to admit anything other than that the cause was "specific, reproductive, and infectious." Incomplete and fragmentary though it was, this work promised much for the future. The consequences of the eventual acceptance of some "germ theory" was not lost on all physicians. In the prophetic words of one such far-seeing medical man: "If such a theory should eventually be proved to be founded on facts, the hypothetical etiology of medical philosophers will be discarded, and medicine be rescued from much of the obloquy which now attaches to it."[46]

The most prominent and consistent of believers in this protogerm theory was Samuel Henry Dickson, professor of medicine at New York University. Convinced since 1832 that cholera was contagious, Dickson had in the seventeen-year interim been supplied with the theoretical arguments to bolster his

---

four years later that favus, a common human skin disease, was also caused by a fungus.

45 *On the Crytogamous Origin of Malarious and Epidemic Fevers* (Philadelphia, 1849). Mitchell states that he has taught such doctrines for years (p. iii). He cites Bassi and others for their work on fungus diseases, though his ignorance of German, he laments, has prevented him "from knowing how far the authors of that country, Henle, Müller, and others have carried their ideas . . ." (p. iv).

Theories similar to that of Mitchell and based on microscopic examination of cholera excreta were advanced in England during the 1849 epidemic and created much interest both in England and in this country. These reports were finally discountenanced by a committee of the Royal College of Physicians, which concluded that the microscopic organisms discovered in the evacuations of cholera patients were not specific for the disease.

46 Robert Southgate, "Medical Sketch of West Point, N.Y., during the Summer of 1849," *New York Journal of Medicine*, IV (1850), 188.

position.[47] The cause of the disease, he decided, though "ultramicroscopic," must be living matter; "whether simply cellular or of complicated structure, whether a fungous sporule or an animalcule, its capacity of self-multiplication, of infinite reproduction, necessarily implies its vitality.[48] Though not certain of their exact nature, Dickson confidently suggested a procedure by which micro-organisms could be proven to cause disease. "*A contagious cell*" was one found only in the animal body when a particular disease was present, and which regularly produced the disease when introduced into the body of another person. Though none of the causative organisms of the great epidemic diseases had as yet been found, Dickson was positive that their natural habitat was the human body.

Most members of the medical profession, however, still regarded the fungoid and animalcular theories as unproven—if not bizarre. Austin Flint, teacher of generations of American physicians, lamented the publication of J. K. Mitchell's treatise on the fungoid origin of disease, for the "author had identified himself with a fanciful hypothesis, which could only serve as a fresh occasion for sarcasm for those who search the annals of medical literature for subjects of ridicule or reproach." Joseph Leidy, the eminent paleontologist and botanist, ridiculed the idea that there could be spores or animalcula in the atmosphere too small to be detected. "It is," he asserted, "only saying in other words that such spores and animalcula are liquid and dissolved in the air, or in a condition of chemical solution." The very idea of looking "for an ague in a mushroom, and for

[47] Dickson had become convinced that cholera was contagious after witnessing an outbreak at isolated Folly Island near Charleston, where the disease had, it seemed to him, obviously been brought by a beached immigrant ship on which the cholera had been raging. Dickson, "On the Communicability of Cholera," *American Journal of the Medical Sciences*, XIII (1833), 359–66.

[48] "On Contagion," *American Journal of the Medical Sciences*, XVIII (1849), 107–18. Dickson does not mention Henle, and it is not clear whether he was familiar with the German scientist's previously published criteria for determining whether a micro-organism caused a disease. It is quite conceivable that Dickson's ideas found their origin in his knowledge of smallpox and vaccination.

a pestilence in a crop of cryptogamous plants" was absurd.[49]

Far more pervasive than any micro-organismic theory, was that which attributed cholera to a "ferment."[50] On what other basis, besides that of personal contagion, could the portability of the disease be explained? (One need only assume that a minute quantity of the "cholera ferment" or "catalyst" had somehow been introduced into a receptive environment.) The atmospheric theory need not be discarded, for it seemed probable that the "fermentation" causing cholera took place in the atmosphere. The same theory might also explain how local nuisances fostered cholera. Fermentation might well evolve a deadly miasm in the dirt, offal, and confined air of urban tenements. Not inherently inconsistent with older ideas, it served to clothe them with the scientific garb necessary in a more critical generation. Nor was the ferment theory inconsistent with the idea that cholera was caused by a micro-organism. Indeed, it was logical to suppose that the ferment might be organic in nature, for only a "nucleated cell," with its indefinite powers of reproduction could "leaven" whole continents.[51]

In no year between 1849 and 1854 was America free of cholera. But then, after 1854, cholera disappeared as abruptly as it had two decades before. It was a dozen years before it was to return.

[49] Flint, *Buffalo Medical and Surgical Journal*, V (1849), 60; Leidy, *A Flora and Fauna within Living Animals* ("Smithsonian Contributions to Knowledge," Vol. V, Art. 2; Washington, 1853).

[50] The works of Liebig were amazingly popular in the United States. By the middle of the 1840's, readers of even the smallest rural weeklies had heard of his work on agricultural chemistry. The interest of American medical men in the so-called zymotic, or ferment, theory of disease seems, however, to have mirrored the interest shown it previously in England.

[51] William MacNeven, "Remarks on the Mode by Which Cholera Is Propagated," *New York Journal of Medicine*, II (1849), 194–95, 201; E. B. Haskins, "Some Remarks on the Febrile Stage of Cholera; with the Suggestion of a New Theory of the Propagation and Spread of Cholera," *Western Journal of Medicine*, III (1849), 384; A. B. Palmer, "Observations on the Cause, Nature, and Treatment of Epidemic Cholera," *Peninsular Medical Journal*, I, 339.

PART 3

1866

X. AMERICA AFTER THE WAR

In the fall of 1865, Americans could for the first time in five years look forward to a peaceful new year. The Civil War had ended; the union had been preserved. Yet the nation which emerged after four years of war seemed to many Americans sadly altered. No longer was the United States immune to the vice and hardship of the Old World.

Nowhere did the departure from older standards seem more apparent than in the cities. The inhabitants of the city's tenements were ignorant of traditional American ways, ignorant in many cases even of English. Still more alarming to pious Americans was their seeming lack of acquaintance with the simplest principles of religion and morality. Crowded slums were, moreover, the source of physical as well as spiritual danger. This conviction, though hardly novel, was becoming increasingly meaningful. Typhoid, dysentery, pneumonia, and tuberculosis were normal hazards of tenement life. In epidemic years, disease claimed an even more disproportionate number of victims from among the city poor.

And 1866 promised to be such a year, for cholera had again swept through Europe. England, France, and Germany had each suffered severely in the summer of 1865; and mere good fortune had kept the disease from American ports in the chaotic months following Appomattox. Having been spared until the fall, Americans could rely upon the cold of winter for protection. Few doubted, however, that another spring and summer could pass without cholera having visited North America.

Yet it need not take its accustomed toll. Science had, in the years since 1849, shown how cholera might be prevented; it was the duty of thoughtful Americans to see that it was. The injunctions of medicine had in the few months before spring to be embodied in statutory law.

The Civil War had intensified, not arrested, America's material progress. The signs were everywhere. Equally apparent to moralists were the spiritual dangers of such rapid progress.[1] Wealth seemed to have become the sole standard of success. Breeding, intelligence, education counted as nothing against its possession.[2] The "reconstruction now most urgently demanded," one editor concluded, "is that of conscience and of law throughout the country." Though the premonitory signs were visible to the moralists many years before, the Civil War seemed to mark a period in America's spiritual life; pious and respectable Americans could not help but express their dismay.

The blood of the people is pulsing quite too fast for health and safety. We are drifting sadly, terribly away from the old landmarks and from every beacon of sense and security. What madness has seized upon the people? How far are these things to carry us?[3]

Although materialism and immorality could be found in the most remote hamlet, it was in great cities that such poisonous growths flourished most luxuriantly. No moralist doubted this observation. New York alone supported thirteen theaters and

[1] Not that the Bible frowned on enterprise. On the contrary, it favored "true progress." But such progress was steady and comparatively slow, "not the flush of fever, the madness of speculation." *Pioneer* (St. Paul, Minn.), August 17, 1866.

[2] See, for example, *Methodist* (New York), VII (April 28, 1866), 132, and the *Hebrew Leader* (New York), January 26, 1866, for two very similar jeremiads from two very different sources.

[3] *Round Table*, III (June 2, 1866), 344.

some two thousand houses of ill fame. So debased an environment offered constant temptation to all but the strongest in faith. The most innocent living in the city's tenements were forced unavoidably into intimate contact with the most depraved.

The population which teems and ferments from cellar to garret into huge tenement houses has been for years absorbing a large proportion of the former middle-class of society, subjecting them to all the lamentable evils which surround such homes. . . . In the tenement house, the virtuous but unfortunate seamstress finds herself on the same floor with lewd women; the honest, but poor mechanic, is in the next room to the burglar on one side and the typhus fever case on the other.[4]

Public-spirited clergymen naturally mentioned the burglar and the typhus case in the same breath, for the physical evils of tenement life were becoming as real to this generation of Americans as its moral hazards had been to their parents. Just as the Young Men's Christian Association was a response to the moral pitfalls of the city, so the public health movement was the result of a growing consciousness of the physical dangers of city life. The increasing use of mortality statistics provided new support for a traditional faith in the healthfulness of rural, as opposed to urban, life.[5] An infant born in the pure air of a

[4] *Christian Intelligencer* (New York), February 1, 1866. The image of a population "teeming and fermenting" is particularly significant, illustrating at once the pervasiveness of scientific ideas and the feeling of distance and inhumanity with which the middle classes regarded the slum dwellers. Equally significant is the expression of fear that the middle class was being proletarianized.

[5] Probably the most widely read of the early uses of comparative mortality statistics in the English-speaking world was that by C. Turner Thackrah, a Leeds surgeon, in his pioneering study of health conditions in his native city, *The Effects of Arts, Trades, and Professions, and of Civic States and Habits, on Health and Longevity* . . . (2d ed.; London, 1832). The most influential of such early American statistical studies was that by Lemuel Shattuck in the famous Massachusetts Sanitary Commission Report that ordinarily bears his name, *Report of the Sanitary Commission of Massachusetts* (Boston, 1850), pp. 82–83. This has been conveniently reprinted in facsimile with a foreword by C.-E. A. Winslow (Cambridge, 1948). The Thackrah study has been reprinted as well, with a foreword by Alexander Meiklejohn (Edinburgh, 1957).

farm or village could expect to live years longer than the child forced to breathe the city's polluted atmosphere. "From the neglect of sanitary precautions, two hundred years ago, the cities would have become depopulated, if it had not been that they were constantly renovated by new blood from the country."[6]

Perhaps the aspect of city life most alarming to mid-nineteenth-century Americans was the increasing gulf which it fostered between rich and poor. In this growing estrangement lay a threat not only to the bodies and souls of individuals, but to the stability of American society. The old bonds of common tradition, origin, and religion seemed to be disappearing. With these ties gone, there was little to protect America from the class hostility and class warfare that convulsed the Old World. New York already rivaled Paris and London in the extremes of splendor and squalor that it harbored.

A thorough grounding in the teachings of religion and morality was the most important requirement in the preparation of a citizen for participation in a democracy. Few Americans would even have thought to question this belief in 1866. Unfortunately, the city poor seemed almost completely alienated from religion and its teachings. The evangelical churches had in the cities become rich men's churches, churchgoing a practice limited to those who could afford pew rent and fine clothing.[7] Where the poor were not completely neglected,

6 New York State Metropolitan Board of Health, *Annual Report . . . 1866* (New York, 1867), p. 11.

7 How, a hard-working mechanic was quoted as remarking, "can I afford to be a Christian and hire a pew and dress up my family in such a style on Sunday that they won't be snubbed for their shabby appearance by genteel Christians?" *Boston Investigator*, XXXV (May 23, 1866), 20. Though the *Boston Investigator* was an anticlerical publication, it said nothing that was not corroborated in the laments of the orthodox. Cf. "A Layman," *Zion's Herald* (Boston), July 25, 1866. The "official" content of American morality and social attitudes was, on the whole, set by the assumptions of these "evangelical churches" (or "orthodox" churches, as religious liberals were more likely to call them). The alienation of the city poor from those values meant—to the members of these churches—their alienation from that which was distinctly American.

wrote a Chicago Presbyterian, they were favored with a variety of attention so condescending that its acceptance humiliated its recipients and merely intensified their hostility to organized religion.[8]

The poor had, in the eyes of pious Americans, become a class without religion. And without it, they were, like the lower classes in European cities, outside society. This lack of piety among the urban poor helped to confirm the widely held assumption that poverty was no accidental condition. If, as critics protested, the Protestant churches had segregated themselves from the masses, it was solely "by virtue of the habits which religion inculcates and cherishes."[9] On the other hand, the exclusive pretensions of the well to do toward piety as well as respectability resulted, naturally enough, in the poor regarding religion with some of the same hostility they did the man of wealth.

The difficulties of bringing religion to the city poor were discouraging even to the most optimistic. In New York, for example, there were some two hundred thousand children between the ages of five and fifteen; and of these, one hundred and twenty-five thousand were estimated to be "unreached and uncared for, as far as moral and religious training is concerned . . . heathens in the midst of a Christian city."[10] Even the most careful rural upbringing might not be proof against the city's blandishments. Few youths maintained church ties after moving to the city to make their fortune, and opportunities for sin were everywhere. As Bishop Simpson of the Methodist Church remarked in an appeal for funds to establish a mission

[8] *North-Western Presbyterian* (Chicago), April 28, 1866. In a smaller community, it was argued, the rich and the poor, the refined and the uneducated were all needed to make up a congregation. In great cities, however, the wealthy and cultivated were numerous enough to form their own churches, and thus deprive their less fortunate brethren of financial and moral support.

[9] *Christian Advocate* (New York), February 8, 1866. "This tendency of things," the clerical editor continued significantly, "is natural and universal, and its results unavoidable; perhaps, we might add, also, not undesirable."

[10] *Advocate and Guardian*, XXXII (January 16, 1866), 20–21.

in New York, there were as many grogshops as there were
Methodists in the city. (Ten thousand to be exact.)[11] The only
religion that flourished in the slums of the great cities was one
as alien as the tenement dwellers themselves.

The poor had been left almost exclusively to the Church of
Rome. In the words of one Catholic spokesman, "the poor
are emphatically here, as they have been always and everywhere, our inheritance."[12] There were few Protestant
churches, he continued, in the lower part of Manhattan Island,
though the less congested—and more prosperous—upper wards
were well supplied. Those of the poor and uneducated not
guided by the teachings of the Catholic church were, he observed, supremely indifferent to everything but the basest of
material considerations. The situation was little better among
Protestants of wealth and education, he concluded, for few ad-
hered with piety or consistency to any particular doctrine.

Judging by the general tone of dismay among Protestant
spokesmen, there was much truth in these strictures. Religion,
as an Episcopal churchman put it, was being left more and
more "to the women and children, and too generally the female children at that."[13] The businessman's contribution to his
church was becoming exclusively a monetary one.

The Protestant churches had money enough; perhaps too
much, evangelical ministers reflected. History demonstrated
that the church had been richest spiritually when poorest in
material things. As the hostile New York *Herald* (January 9,
1866 acidly commented, piety could hardly be expected to
flourish where the gospel was preached from "richly velveted

11 *Methodist* (New York), VII (January 27, 1866), 27.

12 "Religion in New York," *Catholic World*, III (1866), 381–89. Perhaps
more alarming, the anonymous author continued: "A vast mass of the population is completely outside of the influence of any religious body, or any class
of religious teachers professing to expound revealed truths concerning God
and the future life."

13 *Connecticut Churchman* (Hartford), August 11, 1866. This quotation is
drawn from an editorial bewailing diocesan statistics showing three times
as many female as male communicants.

pulpits of royal edifices." While the benevolent spent vast sums in evangelizing pagans in distant lands, the poor in every American city lived without the word of God.[14]

Even the Methodists, traditionally the church of the mechanic and artisan, boasted few communicants among tenement dwellers. Had the descendants of Wesley lapsed in their duty of ministering to the lower classes? Not at all, replied a Methodist clergyman; the Church had never labored with such classes. Until the past quarter-century, America had never harbored a population as ignorant and debased as that which crowded New York and Boston tenements in 1866. "They are foreigners, and such a mass as even the earlier Wesleyans did not operate upon. They are deeper down and more difficult of access than the miners of Cornwall."[15]

None of the nation's great cities could call themselves truly American.[16] How could they be, when so large a portion of their inhabitants was foreign—and not only foreign, but the least desirable among those Europeans emigrating to this country? Immigrants of means and enterprise left the city behind them, pushed on into the interior, and through their exertions, added to the nation's wealth. The "paupers and idlers, vagabonds, and dangerous characters" among the arriving immigrants, on the other hand, "quarter[ed] themselves in the tenements to increase the taxation and crime of the city."[17] Could a democracy based upon such a citizenry long survive?

The Irish especially could not be expected to function as constructive members of a democratic state. To most Ameri-

[14] See, for example, the representative discussion by the Reverend Charles Woodworth, "Popular Evangelization," *Boston Review*, VI (1866), 477–96, esp. pp. 488–89.

[15] J. Miley, *Christian Advocate* (New York), April 12, 1866.

[16] New York was already regarded as particularly alien. In the words of one editorialist, New York, "with its essentially un-American character and corrupt politics, with its vast population, its wealth and its influence upon the whole country, is a terror to all friends of good morals and wholesome legislation." *American Presbyterian* (Philadelphia), May 24, 1866.

[17] *Christian Intelligencer* (New York), February 1, 1866.

cans, they seemed without question to be "politically, one or two stages behind the whole of the Western world."[18] In terror of their priests and still adhering to the traditions of clan life, the Irish voted docilely at the order of some political chieftain. Few American Protestants harbored any affection for the Church of Rome. And "of all Romanists, the Irish were the most bigoted, superstitious, intolerant, and submissive."[19] The plenary council that convened in Baltimore in 1866 dramatized by its meeting, the traditionally assumed dangers of papal subversion. The year 1866 also marked the height of Fenian agitation for an Irish invasion of Canada. This might be tolerated with the whimsy befitting a quixotic crusade of coachmen and housemaids; not so easily dismissed, especially by northern Republicans, was the part taken by Irishmen in the draft riots of 1863 and, in the spring of 1866, in the Memphis race riots.[20]

The Irish seemed to many Americans a misfortune. But this was not true of all immigrants; Americans had little but praise for the Germans and Scandinavians filling up America's still largely empty Northwest. Not only were they needed, they were thrifty, hard-working, churchgoing—in a word, Ameri-

18 *Nation*, I (September 28, 1865), 391. That the Irish usually were enlisted in the Democracy and that Republicans were most alarmed does not, of course, mean that such fears were necessarily—or consciously—self-serving. For a detailed analysis of Irish participation in and attitudes toward American local politics in this period, see Oscar Handlin, *Boston's Immigrants* (2d ed. rev.; Cambridge, 1959). Handlin suggests that the shared sacrifices of the Civil War tended to bring Irishman and Yankee closer together. I have found little evidence suggesting this, though it may have been the case in Boston.

19 *Christian Watchman* (Boston), February 15, 1866.

20 Compare the indulgent comments on the Fenian agitation in the *Journal of Commerce* (New York), March 10, 1866, with the bitterly hostile editorial, "Murder in Memphis," in the *Christian Watchman* (Boston), May 17, 1866. The usual contact, it must be recalled, between comfortable and articulate Protestant Americans—whose views I am attempting to present—and the Irish was that between master and servant. For a typical comment on the plenary council, see the *Presbyter* (Cincinnati), November 7, 1866.

cans, even if they spoke no English.[21] Few Americans doubted that these industrious folk would be quickly assimilated. "The Teutonic element we may welcome as not only the most intimately akin to our own Anglo-Saxon blood, but most capable of all foreign elements of a quick assimilation, physical as well as mental and social with our native race."[22] The almost unanimous support given the union cause by newly arrived Germans had shown that, unlike the Irish, the ideals of liberty were theirs already.[23] Though individual immigrants might be undesirable, immigration was, in sum, an asset to the nation. There was a whole continent still to be subdued. America offered, in the words of Gordon Bennett's *Herald* (May 6, 1866), "room enough and to spare for all Europe here." More important than the tangible assets that the immigrant might bring with him, were the years of labor which he contributed to his adopted country. The immigrant was an indispensable element in the nation's expansion.

Though perhaps necessary to America's growing industries, the immigrant and his family represented at the same time an increasing problem to the nation's cities. Even if all were constantly employed, all well fed and clothed, there was simply no decent housing available for them—and little immediate prospect of any. The medical profession added its voice to that of moralists in demanding reform; for the annual sacrifices claimed

[21] A Kansas editor, for example, expressed a common opinion among midwesterners when he penned a rhapsodic welcome to the fifteen thousand Norwegians expected to settle that year on the plains. "They are a hardy, honest and industrious race, skilled in agriculture and the mechanic arts, and habituated to labor from earliest youth. They are an immense acquisition, and add largely to the productive wealth of the Country." *Freedom's Champion* (Atchison), June 7, 1866. The more orthodox, however, did fear the Germans as infidels.

[22] *Methodist* (New York), VI (December 16, 1865), 396. It is unnecessary to dwell upon the significance of the deterministic assumption that social behavior was the result of racial—that is, biological—factors. Once formulated, it could easily undershore arguments for immigration restriction as American confidence declined and the character of immigration changed.

[23] The historian's controversy over the extent to which Germans actually supported the Union is not relevant here. What is relevant is that Americans at the time thought their support almost unanimous.

by typhoid and tuberculosis were the consequence of remediable faults in housing and sanitation. The epidemics, moreover, which originated and gained momentum in the crowded slums, spread eventually to cleaner and less crowded areas; the problem of the tenements concerned every city dweller. A solution had to be provided if either the bodies or souls of the city's poor were to be saved.

New York had been crowded in 1849. The city had grown in the seventeen years since then, not only in area, but in depth and height as well. "A new town," in the words of George Templeton Strong, "has been built on top of the old one, and another excavated under it."[24] The dangers of this cramped and unnatural existence were undeniable. In 1863, for example, the death rate in New York's notorious sixth ward—site of the Five Points—was almost three times as great as that of the city as a whole.[25] In 1865, 501,327 people lived in New York's 15,357 tenements. The unsanitary and crowded condition of many of these buildings made periodic outbreaks of typhoid, dysentery, and typhus inevitable. In one house on First Avenue, for example, forty-five of ninety tenants had contracted typhoid or enteric fever during 1865, and of these, eighteen had died. These figures no longer surprised the investigating police surgeon once he had seen the building. It was five stories in height, with a twenty-five-foot front and a depth of forty-five feet. The privies were less than six feet from the house, not connected with a sewer, and in the "worst

24 Allan Nevins and Milton Halsey Thomas (eds.), *The Diary of George Templeton Strong* (New York, 1952), IV, 80, April 26, 1866. For a more detailed discussion of tenement conditions, see Gordon Atkins, *Health, Housing, and Poverty in New York City (1865–1898)* (Garden City, N.Y., 1947); Roy Lubove, "The Progressives and the Slums: Tenement House Reform in New York City, 1890–1917" (unpublished doctoral dissertation, Cornell University, 1960), pp. 1–37; Robert Ernst, *Immigrant Life in New York City 1825–1863* (New York, 1949), esp. chap. v, "Tenement Life," pp. 48–60.

25 Dr. A. N. Bell, "The Economy of Human Life," *Bulletin of the New York Academy of Medicine*, III (1867), 229. The death rate was one in twenty-four in the Sixth Ward, while in the Fifteenth Ward, for example, it was one in sixty.

possible condition."[26] Unfortunately, such conditions were neither atypical nor limited to New York. In Cincinnati, for example, a Board of Health inspection reported a two-story house containing one hundred and two persons, for whom only one privy was provided.[27] America could expect little mercy should cholera be imported in 1866.

The "Atalanta," an English mail steamer, sailed for New York from London on the tenth of October, 1865. She docked at Havre on the eleventh, and took aboard twenty-four cabin and five hundred and forty steerage passengers. When she dropped anchor in New York's lower bay, her master reported sixty cases of cholera and fifteen deaths.

It might have been 1848. Ships had increased in size, their passenger lists had doubled, yet no quarantine had been provided. Both medical and political considerations, however, demanded that the passengers of the "Atalanta" be quarantined. A hospital ship was hastily fitted out and as soon as weather permitted, the passengers from the infected steamer were transferred to it.[28] Though new cases occurred aboard the hospital ship, a bitter December discouraged the disease from spreading to the mainland. New York was safe for the moment. But it was clear that this was only a respite—for the rest of the nation as well as for New York.

Quarantines had never succeeded in containing cholera. Only an efficient and thoroughgoing sanitary reform could, it

---

[26] *Evening Post* (New York), January 6, 1866. A later survey concluded that even where drains had been constructed, they consisted in many cases "simply of surface gutters, by which house slops, not infrequently mixed with urine, and even faecal matter, were conducted across the sidewalks and into the street." In addition, privies were often "mere wells, extending from the upper floors to the cellars, and provided with an opening and seat on each floor, but with no provision for water. . . ." New York State Metropolitan Board of Health, *Annual Report . . . 1866* (New York, 1867), appendix, p. 8.

[27] *Enquirer* (Cincinnati), April 13, 1866.

[28] John Swinburne, "The Cholera as It Appeared at the Port of New York in 1865," *Medical and Surgical Reporter*, XIV (1866), 25–26. Forty-two cases of cholera were to occur on the hospital ship.

seemed, guarantee relative immunity. New Yorkers were quick to point out, however, that the legal custodians of the city's health had neither the training, the powers, nor most important, the inclination to accomplish such a reform. Fortunately, winter's cold provided an opportunity, albeit a fleeting one, to enact the necessary public health program into law. Even without the threat of cholera, however, such legislation was inevitable.

Existing arrangements were intolerable. The city did have a health board to be sure. But it was, the Republican New York *Times* (November 10, 1865) acidly commented, "a Health Board composed of such desperate men, that even now with the cholera knocking at our doors . . . a Democratic Mayor of New York now doubtless considers the cholera the less of two evils, and lets the Board alone." This had been the case for years and concerned New Yorkers had for years been defeated in their attempts at reform. For a decade before 1866, efforts had been made to overhaul the city's antiquated system of public health administration; the *Evening Post* had, at one point, even appealed to Lincoln's Sanitary Commission to undertake the work.[29] Perhaps this was a desperate expedient, but five proposed health bills had already failed in the state legislature.

Despite these setbacks, advocates of public health reform felt a new confidence in the winter of 1865–66. It seemed more than probable that the state legislature would, during this winter session, finally pass a measure to preserve the city's health. The threat of cholera was, of course, the most potent and immediate factor favoring the bill's passage. Equally important was the almost unanimous support offered by respectable New Yorkers; it was a measure which no friend of humanity could fail to endorse.

Even without the threat of cholera, the proposed health bill might well have been enacted. For perceptive New Yorkers

---

[29] Nevins and Thomas (eds.), *op. cit.*, IV, 44, November 5, 1866.

saw with increasing clarity the danger of failing to improve the conditions of tenement life—and not only in the area of public health. Even the most obtuse could not have ignored a symptom of discord as striking as the Draft Riots of 1863.[30] Slum life bred riot as it did disease; and though Americans might differ as to the means of treating the underlying conditions which produced social and physical disease, none could, with good conscience, oppose the principle of sanitary reform. It was hardly surprising that New York's Citizens' Association (an informal group of respectable—and predominantly Republican—Gothamites organized early in the 1860's to promote "honest government") should sponsor a subsidiary Council of Hygiene and Public Health.

A group of New York physicians inspired by the achievement of European sanitarians and appalled by the waste of life in New York's slums determined in 1864 to conduct a sanitary survey of the city. They presented their preliminary results to the Citizens' Association, which then agreed to underwrite a more thoroughgoing survey of the city's sanitary condition. To carry out the survey, the association created the aforementioned Council of Hygiene.[31] With the help of a number of interested physicians, the members of the council immediately set to work. Throughout the summer of 1864, these public-spirited medical men thoroughly explored the twenty-nine sections into which they had divided the city.

Their findings were uniformly discouraging. The nauseating conditions described by Elisha Harris, the author of the

---

[30] It must be noted, however, that the public health reformers did not explicitly connect their endeavors with the traumatic effect of the Draft Riots.

[31] The council's membership included such prominent sanitarians as Elisha Harris, Willard Parker, Stephen Smith and Alonzo Clark. For other accounts of the passage of the Metropolitan Board of Health Act, see Roy Lubove, *op. cit.*, pp. 1–37, and Stephen Smith, *The City That Was* (New York, 1911), pp. 41–42. The achievements of Lincoln's Sanitary Commission during the recently concluded Civil War also provided inspiration, and medical officers trained in sanitary matters during the war often returned to lead local health reform movements.

council's final report,[32] crystallized the already alarmed sentiments of thoughtful New Yorkers. Only a complete overhauling of the city's sanitary arrangements would, it seemed, be sufficient to protect the people's health. With the publication of Dr. Harris' report, it had become almost impossible for Tammany Hall to defend rationally the existing state of affairs.

While the Council of Hygiene had been at work inspecting the city's sanitary condition, another creation of the Citizens' Association, its Council on Law, had been occupied in drafting a model public health act. Though a number of New York's most prominent lawyers served on the council, the proposed board of health bill was drafted by Dorman B. Eaton, a public-spirited young lawyer active for almost a decade in public health reform. The detailed provisions of his carefully worded statute reflected clearly the influence of European discoveries and achievements in the new science of public health. It was his implacably detailed measure that had been introduced and defeated in the state legislature in the spring of 1865. Its unobtrusive shelving could not be repeated in the winter of 1865–66; cholera and the Citizens' Association report had made the proposed health bill a major political issue at Albany's winter session.

Proponents of sanitary reform realized that success could come only in the state legislature. New York's City Council could not be expected to discard a system that provided jobs and contracts for the political faithful. The Republicans, moreover, controlled state politics and the Republican minority in New York City—in many cases, the same respectable folk who were the natural supporters of public health reform—saw in this situation an opportunity of stripping Tammany Hall of valuable patronage. And supporters of the health reform bill could, with some justice, argue that all of the city's most valuable institutions, the Metropolitan Police and Fire Depart-

[32] Citizens' Association of New York, *Report by the Council of Hygiene and Public Health . . . upon the Sanitary Conditions of the City* (New York, 1865).

ments, Central Park, and the Croton Water System, had seen
the light of day in Albany. It was absurd, they charged, for
Democratic leaders to state—as they did—that the state legislature had neither the competence nor the experience necessary
to legislate for New York City.

It was equally absurd, proponents of the bill claimed, to
argue as their opponents did that the city's affairs were of no
concern to the rest of the state.[33] The protection of New York
City's health was the concern of every York Stater, indeed of
every American. For cholera in New York City meant cholera
in Albany and Buffalo, on the St. Lawrence, and inevitably
throughout the Great Lakes and Mississippi Valley. To leave
unchanged the sanitary condition of the great port would con-
stitute criminal neglect. The metropolis must, advocates of
public health reform charged, be forced to observe those scientific principles which alone could "prevent it from becoming
a common nuisance in the social organization."[34] New York
had neither the moral nor the legal right to declare its inde-
pendence of the rest of the state. The bill must pass—and pass
before spring. Should it fail, New York City would "literally
be left to its own destruction." And though the poor might
suffer first, they would not suffer alone.

Not the poor and the vicious classes alone will fall victims to the
coming pestilence, for if the great Cholera-fields that now invite
the epidemic in our city be not cleansed . . . the poisons which
they will breed will infect and kill many persons among the more
favored class.[35]

A properly constituted health board would not only guard
against cholera in 1866, but would lengthen and improve the

[33] Democratic editorialists naturally appealed to the traditional antagonism
of New York workers toward upstate Republicans, whom they characterized
as pious and officious hypocrites.

[34] *Albany Evening Journal,* January 18, 1866.

[35] *Harper's Weekly,* X (January 20, 1866), 35. Similar editorial warnings
appeared regularly in New York City throughout January and February in
most Republican papers.

life of New Yorkers every year. The experience of Paris and
London in Europe, and of Providence and Philadelphia in this
country, had demonstrated the benefits of public health reform.

A proper board of health should consist not of political ap-
pointees, sponsors of the bill affirmed, but of medical men
trained especially for public health work. The best medical
talent in France and England served on the London and Paris
health boards. "A merchant or a lawyer would be as much out
of place, in such a sphere of duties, as would a doctor in the
counting room or at the bar." It was as rational, the *Nation*
argued, to give one's watch for repair to a blacksmith as to
allow politicians to be the guardians of the public health.[36]

The political as well as the physical health of the community
would benefit; every job removed from the purview of politicians made the community a healthier one. Efficiency and
professionalism must ultimately replace opportunism and
"placemanship." The public health bill was a reform in the
"right direction," as the *Evening Post* put it, "towards economy and the concentration of necessary authority in the hands
of competent persons."[37] Especially after the arrival of the
"Atalanta," the pressure for the bill's passage became almost
irresistible. The Union League Club, for instance, appointed

[36] "New York and Cholera," *Nation*, II (January 11, 1866), 40–41.

[37] January 26, 1866. The rhetorical stance assumed by the proponents of
the Metropolitan Health Bill was similar to that of the civil service reformers
and liberal Republicans. Indeed, many of the leaders in the fight for the health
bill, such as Dorman B. Eaton, were also active in the civil service cause. Both
civil service and public health reforms would attract the same sort of "middle-
class" support; at least in New York, the poor were appealed to by neither
the moral nor the intellectual arguments for either cause.

Particularly embarrassing, however, to the Republican supporters of the
bill was the two-month delay in its passage while the two Republican factions
that controlled the state legislature disputed its provisions. The Senate, which
was controlled by the "Thurlow Weed interest" insisted on having the power
of appointing the members of the board, while the partisans of Governor
Fenton (who controlled the House) insisted on their version of the bill—
one which gave the power of appointment to the governor. See *Herald* (New
York), January 8, 1866; *Standard* (Brooklyn), February 17, 1866; and the
comments of the "official" Tammany paper, the *Leader* (New York), January 1, February 3, 10, 1866.

a special committee to appear before the legislature and urge its immediate enactment.[38]

On February 26, the bill finally became law. Titled "An Act To Create a Metropolitan Sanitary District and Board of Health Therein," it ran to some thirty closely printed pages, stating in detail the duties and prerogatives of the board. The Metropolitan Sanitary District embraced New York, Kings, Richmond, Westchester, and parts of Queens counties, while the board created to oversee its sanitary condition consisted of a president (to be appointed by the mayor), four police commissioners, the health officer of the port, and four physicians. Most important, and surprising even to the board's warmest supporters, were the sweeping powers granted it.[39]

They would be needed. New York's streets were almost impassible with a mixture of snow, ice, dirt, and garbage. The more despairing of observers reported that the city had never been filthier. Cholera could be expected to show little mercy to a community that harbored such filth—and in which pigs still helped to clean the streets.

[38] The meeting at which the committee was appointed was held January 18. *Evening Post* (New York), January 29, 1866. Included in the group were such prominent New Yorkers as William M. Evarts, J. W. Beekman, Rev. Henry Bellows, and Joseph B. Varnum.

[39] The board was empowered to both create and administer ordinances relating to the preservation of the public health. The bill itself occupies pages 114–44 in New York State, *Laws of the State of New York, passed at the Eighty-Ninth Session of the Legislature* . . . (Albany, 1866), I, chap. 74. The very length and detail of the act are in themselves significant, a measure of the amount of medical and administrative knowledge accumulated in the thirty years since 1832.

XI. THE METROPOLITAN BOARD
OF HEALTH

The new health board faced a staggering task. Between the twenty-sixth of February and the first warm days of spring the accumulated filth of years had to be removed, a city of almost a million thoroughly surveyed and cleansed. And the organization with which to accomplish these herculean labors existed only on paper.

Yet the situation seemed far from hopeless. Never had New York City possessed so powerful a Board of Health; never had physicians and disinterested citizens enlisted in such numbers to help in preserving the community's health. Perhaps most encouraging was the medical profession's new found confidence. "Exact methods of investigation" used during the epidemics of 1849 and 1854 had shown that the poison causing cholera was propagated in "the diarrhoeal and vomited fluids of infected persons."[1] Were this theory sound, the spread of cholera could easily be checked.

And it was, for cholera in New York was limited to a comparative handful of cases. The argument for reform in public health could not have been stated more effectively.[2] The or-

[1] New York State Metropolitan Board of Health, *Annual Report . . . 1866* (New York, 1867), p. 204 (appendix).

[2] It is, of course, doubtful that the mildness of New York's cholera epidemic was due entirely, or perhaps even partially, to the efforts of the Metropolitan Board. The historian, however, must deal with the felt reality of the time, and the fact was that Americans credited the board with having saved the city.

ganization and achievements of the Metropolitan Board exerted a lasting influence; in the history of public health in the United States, there is no date more important than 1866, no event more significant than the organization of the Metropolitan Board of Health. For the first time, an American community had successfully organized itself to conquer an epidemic. The tools and concepts of an urban industrial society were beginning to be used in solving this new society's problems.

In the summer of 1849, Dr. John Snow, a prominent London anesthetist, published a brief pamphlet, *On the Mode of Communication of Cholera*. Dr. Snow argued that cholera was a contagious disease caused by a poison reproducing itself in the bodies of its victims. This poison was to be found in the excreta and vomitus of cholera patients and, according to Snow, it was these substances that spread the disease, most frequently through a contaminated water supply.[3]

Snow's pamphlet caused no immediate stir. His was one among dozens of hopeful theories published at the time. Anyone could, and many did, compose a fanciful etiology of cholera; the problem was to prove it. Snow, unlike the others, did.

When in 1854, London was again severely visited with cholera, Dr. Snow was prepared to test his theory. Fortunately for his plans, if unfortunately for many Londoners, the city was served by two different water companies, the Lambeth and the Southwark and Vauxhall. By a painstaking correlation of the comparative incidence of cholera in subscribers to the two water companies, Snow was able to show that cholera occurred far more frequently among the users of one company's water. This company, the Southwark and Vauxhall, drew its water from the lower Thames, after it had been contaminated with London sewage, while the Lambeth water was

---

[3] Snow also published his ideas in the *London Medical Gazette*, XLIV (1849), 730–32, 745–52, 923–29. For a useful, if brief, review of the importance of Snow's work, see the introduction by Wade Hampton Frost, in *Snow on Cholera* (New York, 1936).

drawn from the Thames above London.[4] How, Snow asked, could such striking data be explained without assuming that cholera was spread by contaminated water? His results were published in 1855 and soon began to win converts.

The most influential of such converts was the great Munich sanitarian, Max von Pettenkofer. The Bavarian scientist had also been able to demonstrate a connection between water and the spread of cholera. Pettenkofer, however, formulated a theory somewhat at variance with that of Snow. He believed that the excreta of cholera patients was not immediately contagious, but had somehow to develop or "ferment" before it was capable of spreading the disease. This fermentation took place, according to Pettenkofer, in the water in the soil. Thus the prevalence of cholera—and typhoid as well—was dependent upon the level of the ground water in any given locality.[5] Despite this somewhat arbitrary aspect of Pettenkofer's formulation, his was a powerful voice added to that of Snow in warning of the dangers of a contaminated water supply. One might disagree with these ideas, but they could not easily be ignored; if Snow and Pettenkofer were correct, cholera could be easily prevented. (One need only disinfect immediately the bedding, clothing, and excreta of those suffering from the disease.)

When in the spring of 1866, the United States was again threatened by cholera, these ideas had been current in medical

[4] Both companies distributed their water generally throughout London; the only variable seemed to be the source from which they drew their supply. More striking than the work I have outlined was the so-called Broad Street pump incident. Snow traced a localized outbreak of cholera to a pump in Broad Street and seemed to have abruptly checked this local epidemic by having the pump's handle removed. Though more famous, this incident is less significant methodologically than Snow's correlation of comparative case rates with an environmental variable. His monograph is still required reading in many epidemiology courses.

[5] There is no satisfactory study of Pettenkofer. Useful, especially for its presentation of his so-called *grundwasser* theory, is *Max von Pettenkofer*, by Edgar Erskine Hume (New York, 1927). Pettenkofer believed that a specific germ or poison caused cholera, though he did not believe that an epidemic could take place unless soil, seasonal, and climatic conditions were propitious. See Pettenkofer, *Untersuchung und Beobachtung über Verbreitung der Cholera* . . . (München, 1855).

circles for a decade and were widely accepted by American physicians. The New York Academy of Medicine, for example, resolved *unanimously:*

That in the judgment of the Academy the medical profession throughout this country should, for all practical purposes, act and advise in accordance with the hypothesis (or the fact) that the cholera diarrhoea and "rice-water discharges" of cholera patients, are capable in connection with well-known localizing conditions, of propagating the cholera poison; and that rigidly enforced precautions should be taken in every case of cholera to permanently disinfect or destroy those ejected fluids.[6]

By 1866, there were few intelligent physicians who doubted that cholera was portable and transmissible.

The rapid assimilation of these ideas should not be surprising. Many American physicians were readers of European medical journals. A greater number kept abreast through the "eclectic" sections of the better American medical journals.[7] (These consisted of summaries of the more important articles in the major French, English, and by the time of the Civil War, German medical journals.) The ideas of Snow, Budd, and Pettenkofer

[6] The resolution is printed in full in the *Medical and Surgical Reporter*, XV (1866), 54. The clause referring to "well-known localizing conditions," was obviously a necessity if a unanimous vote was to be recorded.

In a sampling of the opinions of one hundred and twenty-eight physicians —not including the vote mentioned above—fifty-five were found to have taken a thoroughly "contagionist" stand, while twenty-one could be considered contingent-contagionists. Fifty-two continued intransigent anticontagionists. Forty-five of the sample accepted a least some of the conclusions of Snow and Pettenkofer, while twenty-two were believers in some variation of the germ theory. It should be noted that Pettenkofer was considered a contagionist by contemporaries, though hisorians have often classified him as an anticontagionist because of his outspoken opposition to some of the earlier and more extreme statements of the bacterial theory of disease causation.

[7] John Shaw Billings, for example, noted in 1876 that so excellent were the "abstracts and notices of foreign works [in the *American Journal of the Medical Sciences*], that from this file alone, were all other productions of the press for the last fifty years destroyed, it would be possible to reproduce the great majority of the real contributions of the world to medical science during that period." *A Century of American Medicine, 1776–1876* (Philadelphia, 1876), p. 333.

were no more distant than the nearest post office.[8] Immigrant physicians provided another source of knowledge; in Cincinnati, St. Louis, and New York such men were leaders in advocating contagionism. By settling in these opinion-forming urban centers, a few emigrees might exert an influence far out of proportion to their numbers. So rapid, indeed, was the assimilation of Snow's work in the eastern United States that as early as the summer of 1855, his principles were being applied in the administration of the New York State quarantine hospital.[9]

But opponents were still numerous in 1866. Cholera might be portable, but it certainly did not seem to be contagious in the manner of smallpox or syphilis. Older men, like John H. Griscom, Edwin Snow, and Henry G. Clark, who had spent decades in fighting filth—and who had come almost instinctively to oppose contagionist arguments—could not easily accept a doctrine which promised to destroy the rationale of their work. If, and the argument is implicit in their writings, cholera was contagious and not caused by accumulations of filth, then why need streets and houses be cleaned? Commercial interests also found these new ideas—and the rigid quarantines they implied—unpalatable. When William Read, resident physician of Boston, announced his conversion to the "Snow-Pettenkofer" theory of cholera's transmission, he was quickly reprimanded for espousing doctrines "detrimental to the health, happiness and pecuniary interests of the citizens at large."[10]

Now, however, the epidemiological anomalies that had em-

[8] At least one older physician could not conceal his disdain for "some of our young medical men, who take their medical opinions from the last London periodicals, as the chameleon his hues from the colour of the last branch on which he has basked. . . ." Richard D. Arnold, *Letters of Richard D. Arnold, M.D., 1808–1876*, ed. Richard H. Shryock (Durham, N.C., 1929), p. 130. By the spring of 1866, it is safe to say, any medical man accustomed to even glancing at a medical journal would have come across some mention of the work of Snow and Pettenkofer.

[9] New York State Metropolitan Board of Health, *op. cit.*, p. 217 (appendix).

[10] Read, *A Letter to the Consulting Physicians of Boston* . . . (Boston, 1866), p. 5.

barrassed contagionists in past epidemics could be explained. Knowing that cholera might be spread through a water supply or carried by seemingly healthy persons, the followers of Snow and Pettenkofer were able to discover in the progress of the epidemic further justification for their convictions. Its transmission by human beings, they asserted, seemed too apparent to admit of doubt; in Chicago, the outbreak of the disease was traced to a Mormon immigrant; in Pittsburgh, a few seemingly spontaneous cases on the outskirts were all eventually traced to contacts inside the city.[11]

The common people, of course, continued in their unchanging belief that cholera, like all pestilences, was contagious. Mobs were still one of the normal operating hazards of cholera hospitals. But now, the theories of Snow and Pettenkofer, rather than ozone and electricity as in 1849, were urged upon their readers by newspapers and magazines. Contagionism had become respectable.

Naturally, most physicians, as well as laymen, confounded the ideas of Snow and Pettenkofer with each other, as well as with other concepts, older and more accustomed.[12] Many physicians able to espouse these newer ideas continued to assign a role to the atmosphere in the spread of the disease, while belief in predisposing causes continued to be almost universal—regardless of any other ideas a medical man might entertain. One Yankee physician, for example, who cited Pettenkofer, Snow, and Budd could also marshal an imposing catalogue of predisposing causes, among them "lewdness," and remark that after an epidemic had broken out, an "infection pervaded the air." Other physicians believed that the cholera evacuations had an "infective" or "zymotic" quality only in an atmosphere contaminated with exhalations from decomposing organic matter.

[11] T. Bevan, "The Recent Epidemic of Cholera at the County Hospital, Chicago, 1866," *Chicago Medical Journal*, XXIII (1866), 450–59; Thomas J. Gallagher, "Report of the Allegheny County Medical Society," *Transactions of the Medical Society of Pennsylvania*, 1867, p. 202.

[12] The lingering of predisposing causes and its connection with religious and moral motivations will be treated at greater length in the next chapter.

(Or perhaps, as many felt, a contaminated atmosphere—as in a tenement—must weaken the "system" generally and thus predispose it to cholera.)[13]

Many doctors who accepted the notion that human excreta had something to do with the spread of the disease, failed to understand that these evacuations could spread cholera only if they contained a specific organism or poison. "It has been supposed," wrote one California physician, "that fecal discharges, under some circumstances, favor the production of cholera—especially those from patients suffering with the disease." A New Orleans doctor agreed with the general opinion that cholera was spread through excreta. "But," he cautioned, "not to the extent that many represent. It has to be concentrated and confined."[14] It was still difficult for many medical men to grasp the idea that a specific disease could be caused only by a specific poison or micro-organism.

But new habits of thought, perhaps less conspicuous, betokened the future. Arguments based on formalistic philosophical assumptions almost ceased; statistics and disciplined observation were replacing abstract reasoning. (The imperfections which marred this early work do not invalidate the importance of a newly felt need to perform it.) Contingent-contagionism could, for example, no longer be dismissed as "unphilosophical." Perhaps most striking was the almost unquestioned assumption that cholera was a specific disease. One heard almost

[13] Linus P. Brockett, *Asiatic Cholera* . . . (Hartford, 1866), pp. 62, 96, 99–103, 144–46, 175, 185. The International Sanitary Commission, for example, which met at Constantinople in 1866 and reported unanimously in favor of the idea that the cause of cholera was reproduced in the body of the sufferer, also resolved that "the principle of cholera . . . is volatile, and acts in this respect after the manner of miasma; that is to say, by infecting the atmosphere." International Sanitary Conference, *Report . . . of a Committee from That Body, on the Origin, Endemicity, Transmissibility and Propagation of Asiatic Cholera*, trans. Samuel Abbott (Boston, 1867), pp. 24, 38, 40, 94–95.

[14] H. Gibbons, "Hygiene of Cholera," *Pacific Medical and Surgical Journal*, VIII (1865), 243; Warren Stone, "Cholera and its Treatment," *New Orleans Medical and Surgical Journal*, XIX (1866), 17.

nothing of "universal bowel complaints," of diarrhea "shading into cholera," of cholera transforming itself into typhus.[15]

The assumption that cholera might be caused by micro-organisms met with a mixed, though promising, reception in the United States. Twenty years of scientific advance had made this idea seem less bizarre than it had in 1849. Popular alarm, for example, over the "trichina disease" was at its height in the spring of 1866; and even those who opposed the idea that "mere worms" could cause such a serious illness frequently were led to argue that such parasites were simply normal inhabitants of the human body.[16] The work of Pasteur, moreover, on fermentation and spontaneous generation was becoming known to the general public.[17]

But let us not destroy our understanding through hindsight. Physicians believing in some sort of "germ theory" were still in a small minority—roughly one in seven—while their ideas were crude and inconsistent. But they were listened to; they could no longer be dismissed with a few words of casual ridicule. The painstaking studies of Snow and Pettenkofer had provided the epidemiological underpinning for the rapid and natural acceptance in the United States of Koch's discovery of

[15] One might admit the specificity and portability of cholera and still find fault with the theories of Snow and Pettenkofer. The latter, especially, was the object of much criticism. To some, his *grundwasser* theory was nothing more than an "irreconcilable absurdity." Cholera had spread in the frozen snows of Russia and in the deserts of Arabia. It had made its appearance in places where there could not have been the slightest trace of subsoil filtration. It had prevailed in a citadel perched on the top of one thousand feet of solid rock, while the city at the foot of the mountain escaped. Many other critics emphasized the inability of Snow or Pettenkofer to explain the "isolated cases" that had occurred.

[16] For representative expositions of the "trichina disease," see the *Advocate* (Green Bay, Wis.), April 26, 1866; *Republican* (Chicago), April 14, 1866; *Christian Register* (Boston), March 31, 1866; *Journal of Commerce* (New York), March 26, 1866; *Sunday Dispatch* (New York), February 11, 1866.

[17] See, for example, "W," in the *Zion's Herald* (Boston), July 4, 1866. Illustrative of the lag between scientific advance and popular assimilation of such progress is an unsigned article in the *New York Times*, March 12, 1866, which significantly enough calls the organisms that cause cholera and upon which Pasteur had been working "insects."

the cholera vibrio (1883). As early as 1869, even a firm believer in miasmas had to concede that he was "very fond of the
cell theory" and to predict that there was "more truth to be
developed from that idea than from any other view before the
public mind."[18]

The most compelling of arguments for the organic causation
of the disease rested on the assumption that only living things
had the power of indefinite reproduction, while epidemiological evidence indicated that the cause of cholera was some
specific and infinitely reproducible poison. Though no chemical or microscopic analysis had as yet discovered such minute
organisms, "yet their existence cannot be denied, or we must
admit that these diseases can exist without a cause."[19] The rapid
transmission of the poison and the lethal effect which could be
produced by the ingestion of a very small quantity also implied
that it had the power of reproduction and was, therefore,
organic.

Still, few American physicians were willing to accept
wholeheartedly such theoretical considerations; fewer still
were capable of understanding them completely. Of greater
interest to most American medical men in 1866 were the practical recommendations of Snow and Pettenkofer. Boiling
drinking water or disinfecting clothing and bedding were
measures that any alert physician or board of health could
carry out. At least there was no harm in trying.

[18] Remarks of Dr. John O. Stone at a meeting of the New York Academy
of Medicine, February 11, 1869, *Bulletin of the New York Academy of Medicine*, III (1869), 396 ff.

[19] W. S. Haymond, "The Collapsed Stage of Cholera," *Transactions of the
Indiana State Medical Society*, 1867, p. 101. For similar arguments emphasizing
the necessity of assuming that the cause of cholera was microscopic and
organic, see William Schmoele, *An Essay on the Cause . . . of the Asiatic
Cholera and Other Epidemics* (Philadelphia, 1866), pp. 17–20; J. M. Toner
and Charles A. Lee, "Facts and Conclusions Bearing upon the Questions of
the Infectious Character of Asiatic Cholera," *Medical Record*, I (1866), 201–5;
Henry Hartshorne, *Cholera: Facts and Conclusions . . .* (Philadelphia, 1866),
pp. 46–47.

Cholera had never traversed Europe without subsequently visiting the United States. American men of affairs, and especially those with some interest in medical matters, felt as apprehensive in the fall of 1865 as their counterparts had in 1832 and 1849. Each vessel arriving from Europe that summer and fall brought news of cholera's further spread. Late in the year, the disease established itself in the West Indies. With cholera in the Western Hemisphere, there seemed little likelihood that North America would escape unscathed.[20]

On the first of September, Secretary of State Seward forwarded copies of letters from the surgeon-general and the American minister in Constantinople to the governors of the several states. The ambassador's letter described the epidemic and reported that medical opinion considered it contagious; and without hesitation, the surgeon-general in his covering letter urged state executives to establish "rigid quarantines."[21] Throughout the fall and winter medical societies and local boards of health held meetings and drafted recommendations; what community could consider itself prepared to face a visit from cholera? The editor of the *Boston Medical and Surgical Journal*, for example, observed that the city's sanitary condition was even worse than it had been in the disastrous summer of 1849. "The arbitrary measures," he concluded, "which were then used are imperatively called for now, immediately."[22] New York, as we have seen, the city with most to fear, was foremost in efforts to find a solution to her public health problems.

[20] Fear of the impending epidemic was not as intense as it had been in 1832 and 1849 for the recently concluded war still filled newspaper columns and the public mind.

[21] E. Joy Morris was our minister at Constantinople and C. H. Crane, the acting surgeon-general. Vermont, *Documents Communicated to the General Assembly by His Excellency the Governor, Concerning the Spread of Asiatic Cholera . . . October 19, 1865* (Burlington, 1865).

[22] LXXIII (September 28, 1865), 187. For the preparations of other cities, see, for example, Detroit Board of Health, *Report of a Special Committee . . . Suggesting Measures for the Prevention of Asiatic Cholera . . .* (Detroit, 1865); E. L. B. Godfrey, *History of the Medical Profession of Camden County, N.J.* (Philadelphia, 1896), pp. 94–95.

The Metropolitan Board of Health came into existence on February 26. Within three weeks the board had found quarters, chosen a staff, and issued its first orders. Such speed seemed almost a necessity; the task upon which they had embarked was enormous and the time in which to accomplish it discouragingly short.

Merely cleaning the streets presented a monumental challenge. Every street and court in the city lay, in the words of the *Evening Post*, beneath an accumulation of filth so great that their level was as high above the original grade as the streets of Rome were above the Forum.[23] The board issued its first orders on March 14.[24] By the twenty-third of that month it had investigated and confirmed 2,184 complaints of nuisances and had issued orders against them as "dangerous to life and detrimental to health." The number of such orders had reached 4,343 by the tenth of April and 7,600 by the first of May.

Such determined and vigorous activity implied careful organization. Fortunately for the board, its administrative problems were immeasurably lightened by the co-operation of the metropolitan police. Not only did police officials offer the use of office space, they organized as well a special "sanitary detail" of picked officers to help in enforcing the board's decisions. The police telegraph and messenger service were also at the board's disposal. Each police precinct, moreover, maintained a "complaint book" in which the complaints of private citizens could be made. (Such communication, if signed, could also be made by letter or directly to the board's Central Office.)

23 March 9, 1866. At the risk of seeming either perverse or redundant, let me emphasize again the fact that environmental sanitation was still considered the primary duty of the Board of Health, despite the acceptance of Snow's work. An "energetic" and "active" Board of Health was one that succeeded in keeping the streets clean.

24 The material in this paragraph is extracted from the manuscript minutes of the Metropolitan Board of Health, now in the care of the secretary of the New York City Department of Health. Metropolitan Board, Minutes, March 14, April 10, May 1, 1866. The number of cease and desist orders issued by the board had reached 18,150 by July 20, 1866.

At the end of each day, the complaints were forwarded to the office of the Sanitary Superintendent. Here they were recorded and sorted, and then sent to the sanitary inspector into whose district they fell.[25] It was only after he had investigated and confirmed the reported nuisance that the Metropolitan Board issued an order against it.

Originally it had been thought that one sanitary inspector could without assistance oversee each of the roughly ten-square-block districts into which the city had been divided. (The sanitary inspectors were all physicians, though the law did not specify that they must be.) It soon became apparent, however, that their task was too great; on March 30, the Metropolitan Board resolved to hire assistants for the sanitary inspectors.[26] With their appointment, the board could call upon an unprecedentedly large and well-trained staff—at least for an American board of health. With the active co-operation of the police, and aided by the efforts of many alarmed New Yorkers, the board's workers were able to accomplish much in a short time. One Democratic paper, for example, at first critical of the new health board, observed within a month of its having begun work that the Metropolitan Board had already removed filth sufficient to have made a dozen cities intolerable.[27] Nevertheless, there was still much to be done.

In at least one area, however, the board's efforts had met with little success—it had been unable to arrange for quarantine facilities. New York had had no permanent arrangements since 1858, when an indignant mob had burned the city's quarantine buildings on Staten Island. The "Falcon," hastily fitted up as a hospital ship in the fall of 1865, was the board's only re-

---

[25] Metropolitan Board of Health, *Annual Report . . . 1866*, p. 6 (appendix).

[26] Metropolitan Board of Health, Minutes, March 30, 1866. These clerks, so-called, were to be paid one hundred dollars a month, a respectable salary for the time. Their appointment, however, was only temporary.

[27] *Standard* (Brooklyn), April 14, 1866.

source.[28] Despite its active and enlightened policy, the board and its president, Jackson Schultz, were unable to overcome popular opposition; ordinary folk objected to being exposed to what they had always regarded as contagious ailments.

This need for quarantine facilities was not long in making itself felt. Late in the afternoon of April 18, the steamship "Virginia" dropped anchor in New York's lower bay. Thirty-seven of her passengers had succumbed to cholera on the voyage and another lay dying. There were only fourteen cabin passengers aboard the "Virginia," and her 1,080 steerage passengers were presumed to have been exposed to the disease.[29] More such infected ships could be expected to arrive, and a permanent quarantine would eventually have to be established.

Cholera had appeared in New York harbor with the first warm days of April; it had been well sown in the fall. Despite the admirable efforts of the new Board of Health, few New Yorkers expected their city to escape unharmed. Six weeks of work, however thorough, could not undo the neglect of years.

Cholera claimed its first victim on the first day of May. Another case was reported on the second, and four days later, a third. Ominously, the three victims lived in widely separated parts of the city. George Templeton Strong, like many other New Yorkers, was dismayed. With such sparks scattered throughout the city, it would not be long before they encountered fuel sufficient to start a general conflagration; there were too many tenement houses like that on Mulberry Street in which the second cholera case had occurred, "a nasty overcrowded Irish pigsty."[30]

[28] Since 1858, it had been the practice to detain immigrants on board the ships that brought them. Sick passengers might be transferred to a hulk anchored in the lower bay. The board, enlisting the aid of the emigration and quarantine commissions made a number of attempts to acquire an appropriate tract of land for a quarantine station, but was at first unsuccessful. New York State Metropolitan Board of Health, *Annual Report ... 1866*, p. 53-54.

[29] *Evening Post* (New York), April 19, 1866.

[30] Allan Nevins and Milton Halsey Thomas (eds.), *The Diary of George Templeton Strong* (New York, 1952), IV, 81, May 3, 1866. The condition

With the discovery of the first case on Ninety-third Street, the board immediately set in motion prearranged plans to prevent the disease's spread. At the order of Elisha Harris, the bedding, pillows, old clothing, and utensils—anything that might "retain or transmit evacuations of the patient"—were piled in an open area and burned. Chloride of lime was generously strewn through the house, and five barrels of coal tar and other disinfectants distributed so as to cover the surrounding area.[31] The building was quickly evacuated and its inhabitants moved to hospital tents. For the moment, and to the surprise of most New Yorkers, the disease disappeared.

The next case did not occur until the fourth of June; it was followed by a score of others before the month's end. As yet, however, New Yorkers showed little signs of panic. The cases were scattered, few in number, and limited largely to the filthier parts of the city. There was no explosion of cholera similar to those that had taken place in 1832 and 1849. The mildness of the epidemic was no mere stroke of good fortune, observers agreed, but the result of careful planning and hard work by the new health board.

As soon as they were chosen, the board's medical advisors had begun to draft plans. There was little enough time before spring and cholera's almost certain appearance. The Battery Barracks were secured from the secretary of war for possible use as a hospital (though a cordon of police had to be provided to protect the barracks from violence). Another building was procured for storage of the chemicals to be used in disinfection of the excreta and personal effects of cholera vic-

of the house at 115 Mulberry Street seems to have been particularly disgraceful. The rooms were tiny, and some of the residents of the five-story building were forced to board up their windows because of the odor rising from the filth deposited in the narrow airshafts separating theirs from adjoining buildings. "Add to this the custom borrowed from untutored animals confessedly low in the scale, of depositing faeces in the halls, and the picture of this haunt of the lowly may be pronounced complete." *Medical Record*, I (May 15, 1866), 151.

31 *New York Times*, May 2, 1866; *Evening Post* (New York), May 2, 1866.

tims. A number of wagons were purchased; and these, together with a sufficient complement of horses, were kept in a stable close by. Also quartered nearby and in constant readiness were details of men specially trained in the use of disinfectants.

When, on May 1, the city's first cholera death was reported, this plan was put smoothly into operation. Each case was reported at the closest police precinct station. The victim's address was immediately telegraphed to the board's Central Office, which quickly dispatched a wagonload of disinfectants to the infected premises. Within an hour of the original report having been made, a detail of well-trained men would be at work disinfecting the clothing, house, and effects of the victim.

Soon after the board was organized, and well before the city's first case of the disease, an anticholera mixture was prepared and distributed in one-ounce vials to the several precinct houses; they were to be distributed to those of the poor complaining of cholera's premonitory symptoms. With the co-operation of the city's privately endowed medical dispensaries, a "movable corps" was established for house-to-house visitation.[32] Arrangements were made as well for providing with food and clothing those families which might be stricken by cholera. The desperate improvisations of 1832 and 1849 would not be re-enacted in 1866.

Even with its new powers, however, the board was not immediately able to find a solution for all of its problems. Two dilemmas were particularly intractable—the problem of providing quarantine facilities and that of improving the city's sanitation. In the first instance, the board had to oppose traditional fears and, in the second, traditional practice, specifically the contract system of street cleaning and waste disposal. In neither area was the Metropolitan Board completely successful.

But not because of a lack of effort. Judicial injunctions ultimately frustrated the elaborate—and almost ludicrously surreptitious—attempts of the board to acquire and fit out a

[32] New York State Metropolitan Board of Health, *Annual Report . . . 1866*, p. 21 (appendix); Metropolitan Board of Health, Minutes, April 27, 1866.

quarantine hospital. The problem of sanitation was even more annoying. Throughout the spring and summer of 1866, the new board and its preternaturally energetic president, Jackson Schultz, were mired in the seemingly hopeless task of attempting to force the city's contractors to fulfil the conditions of their contracts. (It will be recalled that street cleaning and waste disposal were performed for the city by private contractors.) On the fifteenth of March, for example, at the board's second meeting, President Schultz met with all the contractors; past sins, he conceded, would be ignored if they would carry out their tasks in the future. If not, he threatened, the city would have the work done and charge the expense to the contractor. Such threats and cajoling were repeated again and again, though to no avail. The moral seemed clear; a great city could not depend upon private contractors for the carrying out of such vital tasks. Especially when, as was clearly the case, such contracts were regarded as political rewards rather than commercial obligations.

New York's bench added as well to the board's difficulties. Despite its theoretically almost unlimited powers, the orders of the board were nullified again and again by injunction. This was a decade of understanding judges; the first injunction against the board's activities, for example, was issued by Judge Barnard, whose role in the Byzantine affairs of the Erie railroad has earned him a secure, if small, place in history. A month later, the same justice issued another injunction in the name of a number of Staten Island property owners, enjoining the use of Seguine's Point for quarantine purposes. (Judge Cardozo of the Court of Common Pleas was also prevailed upon to issue injunctions against the enforcement of certain parts of the sanitary code.) Equally handicapping to the board was the court's defeat of its attempts to exercise preventive powers. As interpreted by New York judges, the board's powers extended only to the correction of existing abuses. A health officer might, for example, order a vacant lot cleaned, but, thought it were obvious that the lot would within a week be buried again in filth, he had no power to have a fence erected to prevent it.[33]

Legal obstacles were not the only ones placed in the way of the board; a creation of a Republican legislature, it was consistently opposed by the city's Democratic papers and politicians—at least at first. The board, they charged, was the creation of "rural lawyers," who saw no harm in giving non-elective commissioners such wide executive powers.[34] Once the board had begun its work, it was not difficult for Democratic journalists to convince lower-class readers that the policies of the board favored the rich at their expense. The poor were as unprepared to accept the absolute authority of science as they had been to accept the moral absolutism it was replacing; and it was only by assuming the values of science and accepting its dictates as above dispute that the seemingly authoritarian policies of the health board could be justified. To the editor of the Catholic *Freeman's Journal*, the "In-Sanitary Commission" was "positively a detriment to the health of the city, and a vile annoyance." The board, he charged, had been quick to attack the Washington market—a boon to widows and thrifty boarding-house keepers—but had done nothing about the tenement houses, the real source of danger to the people's health. The physicians attached to the board were not its guiding force, he added, but merely the dupes of the "two or three sharp political swindlers" who employed the authority of science as a cloak for their malefactions.[35]

---

[33] Appendix "F," pp. 358–65, in the *Annual Report* for 1866 of the Metropolitan Board is the report of the board's attorney.

[34] *Leader* (New York), April 14, 1866. Conservative Democrats, who tended to represent circles with greater education and social status, had never opposed the board as violently as had the *Freeman's Journal*, for example. As the spring and summer advanced, their lingering opposition turned to praise. The board was the kind of issue upon which social—and in New York, necessarily ethnic—considerations might take precedence over normal political alignments.

[35] April 21, 26, 1866. Indicative of the class assumptions implicit in the editor's appeals was his attack on the board's announced policy of requiring marriage registration. What, he asked, of the cases in which a marriage certificate must be postdated in order to preserve a woman's reputation? *Freeman's Journal*, May 26, 1866.

These arguments only confirmed the fears of conservative Americans, already feeling misgivings about immigrants and, in a few cases, already questioning the viability of democracy itself. It seemed to them that every step toward efficient and responsible government was opposed by the forces of ignorance and immorality. How, for example, they asked, could one hope to institute a successful public health program among an illiterate and vicious population? European governments could command; Americans must depend upon the enlightenment of the voters and those they elected. Ours was a system of government devised and practiced "by the old American population of fifty years ago, those quiet, thrifty, reading farmers, who laid the foundations of American society, who were for two centuries its boast and glory, and are still its salvation. . . ."[36] Unfortunately, these "reading farmers" were being replaced by people of a very different sort. American democracy would, in their hands, come to be synonymous with "unlimited license, unrestrained brutal indulgence, and the overthrow of every principle which has made American institutions superior to those of other countries."[37]

Opposition to the board's policies was inevitable, its complete success beyond the hopes of its most enthusiastic supporters. The surprises of the board's first year were all pleasant ones. Though New York had greatly increased in size between 1849 and 1866, there were only a tenth as many cholera deaths in the latter year.[38] What stronger testimony could there be to the achievements of this new-model health board?

Even bitter opponents finally admitted that the board had proven itself honest and efficient. A Democratic editor, for example, vigorously opposed to the Metropolitan Board at

[36] *Nation*, II (May 11, 1866), 600–601.

[37] *Christian Intelligencer* (New York), June 7, 1866. "Is democracy henceforth to be the sole creed of the lawless, reckless, disobedient masses . . . ?" asked the troubled editor.

[38] There were only 591 deaths in New York. New York State Metropolitan Board of Health, *Annual Report . . . 1866*, p. 189 (appendix).

first, was forced by September to declare that "if we had had no Health Board we would probably have had a great deal more cholera."[39] Equally significant was the unwilling praise accorded the board's efforts by a homeopathic physician. New York's relative immunity from cholera was, he confessed, "in no small part" due to the Board of Health, for it was undoubtedly efficient, "though as bigoted as the inquisition of old."[40]

There was no denying the immense work it had accomplished. The board had, for the first time, cleaned the city's streets, had even made New York's air a bit more breathable—but not without effort. One of the board's first tasks, for example, was the removal of some hundred and sixty thousand tons of manure from vacant lots. Between the fourteenth of March, when the new health board issued its first cease and desist order, and the first of November, 31,077 such orders were issued and served. Some four thousand yards were ordered cleaned, 771 cisterns ordered emptied, 6,418 privies disinfected.[41] Only by such thoroughgoing labors could a city be protected against disease.

The lesson taught by the Metropolitan Board was a simple one. A board of health had, by its efforts, turned away a cholera epidemic from the largest and most congested city in North America. Medical men and concerned citizens in general throughout the United States called for the creation in their communities of health boards similar to that which was credited with having saved New York.[42] No American city

---

[39] Compare the editorial comments in the *Metropolitan Record*, a violently "Copperhead" publication, on May 19 (p. 15) with those made by its editor on September 8 (p. 2) and July 7 (p. 2).

[40] *United States Medical and Surgical Journal*, II (1867), 210.

[41] New York State Metropolitan Board of Health, *Annual Report . . . 1866*, pp. 18, 26, 38.

[42] Cf. H. Gibbons, *Pacific Medical and Surgical Journal*, IX (1866), 216; Thomas N. Bonner, *Medicine in Chicago, 1850–1950* (Madison, 1957), pp. 180–81; *Enquirer* (Cincinnati), August 9, 1866; *Weekly Missouri Democrat* (St. Louis), July 31, 1866; *Catholic Mirror* (Baltimore), April 7, 1866; J. R. Stevenson, "A History of Cholera in Camden in 1866, and of the Measures Adopted for Its Prevention," *Transactions of the Medical Society of New Jersey*, 1867, pp. 236–37.

possessed a board of health with powers even approximating those of the Metropolitan Board of Health—and few such cities escaped cholera as lightly.

The public concern which had in the spring of 1866 lent urgency to the plans of the Metropolitan Board of Health was not limited to New York. Sanitary commissions and boards of health throughout the nation were created, activated, or refurbished. None, however, were endowed with the broad powers of the Metropolitan Board of Health; none were staffed by medical personnel as competent, energetic, and well informed. In Cincinnati, for example, the Board of Health had managed to keep the streets fairly clean, but was unable to force private property owners to abate nuisances in their houses and yards. The president of Buffalo's Health Board, though a medical man, received a salary of $150 per annum—distressing indication of how demanding his duties were expected to be. Smaller communities were even more casual in their gestures at public health reform. The citizens of Staunton, Virginia, were, for example, reminded that "throwing dirt, dead dogs, cats, &c, on the street any day but Saturday, will subject them to arrest and fine."[43] Staunton was, unfortunately, no more errant than many American towns.

Or large cities. Chicago had no board of health at all; since 1861, the protection of the city's health had been the responsibility of the police department. In Cincinnati, no hospital was provided for cholera patients until the daily death toll reached ninety. It seemed hardly surprising that neither city escaped cholera lightly. The moral was equally clear; in March of 1867, the Illinois state legislature provided Chicago with a board of health modeled closely on that of New York.[44] The

[43] For Cincinnati: "S," *Daily Gazette*, August 9, 1866; for Buffalo: William Gould, "Inaugural Address . . . ," *Buffalo Medical and Surgical Journal*, V (1866), 435; for Staunton: *Valley Virginian*, July 25, 1866.

[44] Chicago's Common Council had, like New York City's local government, opposed the establishment of such a health board. Chicago Board of Health, *Report of the Board of Health of the City of Chicago, for 1867, 1868 and*

entire United States, not only New York, was ultimately to
benefit from the farseeing efforts of those physicians, lawyers,
and reform-minded citizens responsible for the creation of the
Metropolitan Board of Health.[45] Disease could be prevented—
this was the truth made undeniable by the success of the Metropolitan Board of Health. Physicians had tried to cure cholera; 1866 had shown them their duty was to prevent it.

1869; and a Sanitary History of Chicago, from 1833 to 1870 (Chicago, 1871),
pp. 54–55, 57–58, 86–106, 119–20; *Republican* (Chicago), May 5, August 14,
1866.

[45] The details of the statute drafted by Dorman Eaton provided as well
the legal mechanisms through which the inspiration of the board's achievements could be transformed into administrative reality. Stephen Smith, *City
That Was* (New York, 1911), p. 158. Its provisions were copied again and
again in succeeding decades as other American communities created their own
boards of health.

XII. THE GOSPEL OF PUBLIC HEALTH

The Metropolitan Board of Health had shown that cholera could be prevented—not with prayer and fasting, but through disinfection and quarantine. To ministers as well as physicians, government had no greater responsibility than to preserve human life; the gospels of Snow and Chadwick, not those of Mark and John, promised deliverance from cholera.

God was still in his heaven, as most Americans would be quick to affirm. Yet the fact of his existence had ceased to be a central and meaningful reality in their lives. The warnings of perceptive divines in 1832 were proving justified; material preoccupations and empirical habits of thought had not so much defeated as displaced the spiritual concerns of earlier generations. America seemed well on the way toward becoming a land of "practical atheists."

Revolutions in thought are always gradual, however, and older values continued comfortably to coexist alongside the new. Moralism, if not theology or piety, still pervaded medical thought, as it did the American mind in general. Sin, in the scientific guise of predisposition, could still induce a case of cholera. Not until the advent of that converting ordinance, the germ theory, did most physicians completely accept the idea of specific disease entities and begin to make an absolute distinction between physical and psychic maladies.

The American medical profession was in transition in 1866. While medical science had already entered an age of heroic achievement, the practitioner of medicine still occupied much the same lowly status he had in 1849. The critical temper productive of the scientific advances that have so transformed the status of the American physician in the twentieth century served in 1866 merely to underline the profession's real, if transitory, inadequacies.

On October 4, 1865, a group of public-spirited New Englanders met in the Massachusetts' statehouse to found a Society for the Promotion of Social Science.[1] The methods of science could, and must, they felt, be applied to the study of human society. The activities of this new association were to be divided among four "departments," the first three of which (education, jurisprudence, and social economy) represented no novel interests. The fourth, however, was something of a new departure for those interested in social betterment. It was sanitary reform.

Physicians could not help those stricken with cholera. Medicine offered no remedy for smallpox. Yet science had shown that both diseases could be prevented, the one by vaccination and the other through disinfection and quarantine. What, one might well ask, had medicine ever contributed to the sum of human happiness? The answer was all too obvious to those skeptical of traditional remedies: the only real contribution of medicine to civilization was the sanitary and hygienic regulations it had helped institute. Such laws were worth more than all "the drugs of Galen and Paracelsus combined." Not only in the United States, but throughout Europe, cholera demonstrated forcefully that a disease that could not be cured must be prevented. Acting as a catalyst, cholera helped to bring about the creation of the public health reforms demanded by the almost unendurable conditions of the nineteenth-century city.

The statistics gathered by a generation of public health workers had convinced Americans of the necessity for sanitary reform; what objective could take precedence over that of

[1] *Nation*, I (October 12, 1865), 449.

preserving human life?[2] Though cholera might appear once in a generation to destroy thousands of lives, tuberculosis and pneumonia killed as many each year. Fortunately, however, the legislation enacted to prevent cholera would help banish these everyday ills as well. No city could call itself civilized that neglected such mundane matters as sewers, drains, and wells. As Cincinnati's health officer put it:

Before erecting statues, building opera houses and art galleries, and buying expensive pictures, towns should be relieved of bad odours and fermenting pestilence. Good privies are far higher signs of civilization than grand palaces and fine art galleries.[3]

Life itself must be guaranteed to man before one could hope to improve his mind—or his soul.

The clergyman was beginning to accustom himself, as the physician already had, to thinking in environmental terms. "What opportunity is there of benefiting the souls of man," questioned one Methodist preacher, "while their bodies are thus crowded and packed in such filthy abodes?"[4] To experi-

---

[2] During most of the centuries before the nineteenth, of course, such a rhetorical question might well have received the immediate answer, "many." For a discussion of early ideas regarding the prolongation of human life, see Gerald J. Gruman, "A History of Prolongevity Hypotheses to 1800: The Evolution of Ideas about the Prolongation of Human Life," (unpublished doctoral dissertation, Harvard University, 1960).

[3] William Clendenin, *Daily Gazette* (Cincinnati), July 23, 1866.

[4] J. M. Freeman, "New York City as a Mission Field," *Methodist*, VI (December 30, 1865), 409. The connection between man's physical and moral well-being was hardly a novel one. Cf. John Griscom, *The Sanitary Condition of the Laboring Population of New York* (New York, 1845); New York Association for Improving the Condition of the Poor, *First Report of a Committee on the Sanitary Condition of the Laboring Classes in the City of New York* . . . (New York, 1853), pp. 3–4. Particularly revealing in this connection is the position of Jackson Schultz, the president of the Metropolitan Board of Health, in the board's *Annual Report . . . 1866*, p. 11.
His professional contact with disease and poverty often leads the physician toward criticism of the society that allows such conditions to exist. Rudolf Virchow's experiences as a young man in fighting a Silesian typhus epidemic, for example, made the great pathologist a confirmed liberal for the rest of his long life. Erwin H. Ackerknecht, *Rudolf Virchow* (Madison, Wis., 1953). See also George Rosen, "Disease and Social Criticism: A Contribution to a Theory of Medical History," *Bulletin of the History of Medicine*, X (1941), 5–15.

ence, as did the board of health officer or the city missionary, the conditions of tenement life was to discredit moralistic explanations of poverty as well as of disease. Alcoholism, for example, seemed to such environmentally oriented Americans not so much a cause of poverty as a consequence of the misery in which the poor were forced to live. "If you lived in this place," a drunken slum mother bitterly replied to the health officer's inquiries, you too "would ask for whiskey instead of milk."[5]

Material evils demanded material remedies. Disease, for example, could not be conquered until better housing was provided for the poor. If tenements must exist—and there could not be cities without them—they should be as clean and well ventilated as architecture and engineering could make them. The Five Points must be regenerated, one liberal editorialist agreed, but it could not be accomplished with missions or Bible classes: "The remedy of all evils in great cities," he asserted, "must be topographical."[6]

The achievement of municipal and personal hygiene were goals well within the canon of traditional Protestant values. Yet cleanliness was coming more and more to be a real and sufficient good, not merely a symbol of spiritual grace. It was a goal, nevertheless, and one which could for its fulfilment call upon those moral energies accumulated by an earlier generation in its struggle for salvation. Personal cleanliness was urged with an almost transcendent zeal; bathing, for example, promised moral as well as physical rewards:

That horrible class from which come the wretched, the vicious, the depraved, would be sensibly diminished, for the "great unwashed" would exist only in name; the "great washed" would be, in a measure at least, the "great virtuous."[7]

5 New York State Metropolitan Board of Health, *Annual Report . . . 1866*, p. 135 (appendix).

6 *Citizen* (New York), March 31, 1866.

7 Reverend Octavius B. Frothingham, *Universalist* (Boston), May 26, 1866. If temporal matters intruded into the realm of the spirit, spiritual needs displayed on occasion the same sort of imperialism, *vide* Christian Science.

The distinction between the physical and spiritual had become increasingly indistinct.

Christianity defined clearly the duties of the employer toward his employees and of the landlord toward his tenants. With men's eyes fixed on the world around them, the failure to fulfil such responsibilities became ever more apparent—especially in cholera times. Statistics had proven what common sense had already known: in any epidemic, those who had the faintest chance of surviving were those who lived in the worst conditions, in the dirtiest, most crowded, and least ventilated houses. It was clear that men who knowingly allowed such conditions to exist were guilty, in a sense, of murder. If, one editor commented, there was a moral in cholera, it was that the landlord who grew "rich by the misery of the poor, who derives revenue from over crowded tenements and cellar lodging houses is guilty of a crime against humanity and against God."[8]

Science provided not only the appropriate goals for reform, but implied a new strategy for their attainment. Criticism of social injustice might now be couched in pragmatic terms, terms congenial to the moderate aspirations of respectable Americans. Clean and airy tenements, an honest and competent civil service, were goals that readily won the support of the thoughtful and educated. Society as a whole need not be rejected in order to make a better world. Social injustice was simply another problem to be solved. The absolutist frames of reference assumed in 1832 seemed no longer particularly relevant to the needs of most Americans in 1866.

The cholera epidemic, declared George Templeton Strong, "is God's judgment on the poor for neglecting His sanitary laws."[9] To die of cholera was still a sign of moral indiscretion; poverty was still very much a result of moral failings. It was not, as a city missionary put it, "that the poor are invariably ignorant and vicious, or the rich learned and virtuous.

[8] *Standard* (Brooklyn), May 5, 1866.

[9] Allan Nevins and Milton Halsey Thomas (eds.), *The Diary of George Templeton Strong* (New York, 1952), IV, 96–97, August 6, 1866.

We only assert the union here, as in other places, of the three most terrible evils that afflict society—poverty, ignorance, and crime."[10] Such age-old ideas were not easily discarded, despite the century's increasing environmentalism.

In the classifications of formal rhetoric, the poverty of any-one not widowed, or crippled, or feeble-minded was somehow culpable. Wealth, in like manner, was still in most cases the product of industry and intelligence. If it was the duty of the employer to care for his employee, it was equally the duty of the worker to identify himself completely with the fortunes of his employer. Even advocates of public health reform found it difficult to dissemble the instinctive distaste which they felt for the dirty and uncouth slum dweller.[11]

It still seemed natural that cholera should single out such persons for destruction. As the *New York Times* (April 22, 1866) expressed it: "Cholera is especially the punishment of neglect of sanitary laws; it is the curse of the dirty, the intemperate, and the degraded." The three adjectives were closely related and, to most Americans, at once cause and consequence of poverty. To ardent temperance advocates, the banishment of liquor would curb poverty as neatly as it halted cholera.

Nor was there any necessary inconsistency between the ideas that cholera was caused by "dirty water" and that it was provoked by intemperance. One still had to predispose oneself to a disease before it could be contracted. There seemed little reason for most physicians to doubt the importance of pre-disposing causes in explaining the occurrence of cholera; even the most convinced believer in the disease's specificity had somehow to explain why only some of those exposed to its

[10] And this from the same Reverend Freeman, cited earlier (n. 4) for his advocacy of the idea that men's souls could not be saved while they lived in filth. *Methodist*, VI (December 23, 1865), 401.

[11] In New York's slums, for example, wrote the editor of the Albany *Journal* (February 6, 1866) in the course of an appeal for the passage of the Metropolitan Board of Health Act, the visitor would "behold the excess of degradation of which pure animalism is capable, in a grade of humanity which literally wallows like swine in the mire."

specific cause became ill (a problem conveniently ignored in the overeager acceptance of the germ theory during the last decades of the century).

The list of possible predisposing causes had not lengthened greatly in the years since Americans first encountered cholera in 1832. (After all, there are only so many misdeeds one is capable of committing.)

As to what are the exciting causes of cholera, there appears to be no diversity of opinion throughout the medical profession. . . . Those arising from personal condition are intemperance, profligacy, immorality, uncleanliness, fear, sensual indulgence, excessive labor, extreme fasting, innutritious diet, want of sleep. . . .[12]

Yet the espousal of this moralistic etiology was becoming increasingly uncongenial to the more critical among the medical profession. This doctrine seemed to them founded upon Philistinism and moral complacency, not upon the verifiable truths of science. "Must," complained a prominent Cincinnati practitioner, "every poor victim of cholera have written, 'In Memoriam', that he was low Dutch, or low Irish, or intemperate, or licentious or a groveler in filth, or a suicide from imprudence?"[13]

Though a few physicians might argue that cholera was not a specific disease or that it might find its origins in local "exciting causes,"[14] the great majority wholeheartedly accepted the idea that cholera was a specific disease, the result of having imbibed some quantity of a specific poison. Though predisposing causes had, as we have seen, not disappeared from med-

[12] William Read, *A Letter to the Consulting Physicians of Boston* . . . (Boston, 1866).

[13] W. H. Mussey, *Cincinnati Lancet and Observer*, IX (1866), 616–17.

[14] See William B. Fletcher, *Cholera: Its Characteristics, Treatment, Geographical Distribution* . . . (Cincinnati, 1866), pp. 19, 24; M. L. Linton, *Medical Record*, I (1866), 143; Julius Miner, "Reasons for Fearing the Appearance of Cholera in Other Epidemics," *Buffalo Medical and Surgical Journal*, V (1865), 119; *ibid.*, V (1866), 299; N. S. Davis, "How Far Do the Facts Accompanying the Prevalence of Epidemic Cholera in Chicago . . . Throw Light on the Etiology of That Disease?" *Chicago Medical Examiner*, VIII (1867), 646.

ical thought, they had become increasingly an afterthought.[15]

The hand of God was being withdrawn from the world. With each epidemic, the role of the divine in causing cholera had become a smaller one. Even the moralism informing the doctrine of predisposing causes existed tenuously, without either the formal underpinning of theology or the emotional assurance of personal piety; religion was in danger of becoming a social gesture.

Far less than in 1849 did cholera provoke an explicit ideological conflict between scientific and religious ideas.[16] Most clergymen called no longer for fast days and spent little time in asserting God's power of intercession in earthly affairs. Disease was a result of having failed to observe the laws that he had established for the government of the world. "Dirt and degradation are antagonistic to divine law"; men would naturally suffer if they persisted in defying the divine ordering of things.

The familiar arguments of 1832 and 1849 were repeated once again—but with an increasingly secular tone. Only God could give or take away life, true. Yet he co-operated with every attempt to increase man's health and happiness. Vaccination, as one clergyman pointed out, had saved at least four hundred thousand lives in Europe alone during the past half-century. There had been no evidence of divine displeasure at such "impiety." On the contrary, he concluded, "we may reasonably hope that with increasing health will come a nobler opportunity for that holiness which is only the perfect whole-

---

[15] As one might suppose, the more clearly one accepted and understood the newer ideas of epidemiology, the smaller the role one allotted to predisposing causes. Snow, for example, declared that "to be of the human species, and to receive the morbid poison in a suitable manner, is most likely all that is required." "On Continuous Molecular Changes. . . . Being the Oration Delivered at the 80th Anniversary of the Medical Society of London," *Snow on Cholera* (New York, 1936), p. 161.

[16] The lack of precision with which religious and scientific ideas were expressed is, of course, another reason for the surpassing ease with which they were made to dovetail.

ness of body and soul in man, the wondrous immortal child of God."[17]

Fast days were beginning to seem the concern of fanatics. The *Independent* (August 16, 1866), probably the most influential religious paper in the United States, retold with evident relish, for example, the famous anecdote of Lord Palmerston's having refused the request of a delegation from the Scottish Kirk for the declaration of a fast day against cholera, urging them instead to go home and clean their streets. God had commanded us to obey his ordinances, and there were none more important than those which bade us to keep clean and healthy. There was no necessary conflict between the truths of science and those of revealed religion. "Science and Religion may each one shine with a new and peculiar beauty in each other's light; they cannot obscure or destroy one another."[18] Yet skepticism often lurked beneath the cloak of science; piety had more to fear from the subtle skepticism of Darwin and of Buckle than it had from the blatant atheism of a Paine or Volney. Consider, for a moment, the apparently abstract question of spontaneous generation: Were Pasteur's opponents in the right, life might come into being at any time, thus undermining God's unique role in creation. Men of the cloth could not reject these new sciences. Indeed, it was their duty to study them, for the church needed "men who can thread all the windings of scepticism, and wrest the weapons of infidelity to its own destruction."[19]

[17] Reverend A. D. Mayo, *Daily Commercial* (Cincinnati), March 25, 1867, cited in the *Eclectic Medical Journal* (New York), II (1867), 271–74.

[18] *Christian Intelligencer* (New York), January 18, 1866. The "conflict between religion and science," so beloved of historians, has, at least in the United States, been more a class and regional than an intellectual struggle. The evolution controversy, for example, drew its emotional intensity not from the irreconcilable nature of the ideas involved, but from urban-rural and upper-lower class cleavages.

[19] Charles L. Woodworth, "Popular Evangelization," *Boston Review*, VI (1866), 477–96; "W," Boston *Zion's Herald*, July 4, 1866.

The status of the medical professon was, in 1866, not appreciably different from what it had been seventeen years earlier. The average physician was still poorly educated and not overly genteel. Even more important, he was a dispenser of nostrums only a bit less heroic than those prescribed by his teachers.

Educational standards were, if possible, lower. As the operation of a medical school was a source of income, there was little reason for turning away prospective students. Neither a college degree nor, what was far more scandalous for the time, a knowledge of the classics was required for entrance into medical school; the profession, it was clear, made few demands on the student physician's intelligence. Which, lamented the president of the Pennsylvania Medical Society, "is, obviously, a great cause why so many feeble-minded boys are dedicated to its study."[20] Despite the establishment of the American Medical Association's Code of Ethics (1847), commercialism, rivalry, even fraud continued unchecked. (Such desperate competition might be expected in the absence of uniform licensing provisions and at a time when minimal education standards prevailed.) Physicians, like other Americans, were businessmen; the rigid institutional codes traditionally associated with the profession seemed somehow irrelevant.

Yet there had been some changes in medical practice. Most obviously, the physicians' remedies had become somewhat less traumatic.[21] The reasons for this change are several—and illuminating. An obvious reason, of course, was the discouraging experience that Americans had had with cholera. Medicines had shown themselves to be useless, once well-marked symptoms of the disease appeared. Experience had made clear, and by 1866 it was fashionable to report, that those cholera pa-

---

[20] J. D. Ross, "Address of the President," *Transactions of the Medical Society of Pennsylvania*, 1865, p. 30.

[21] A study of prescriptions in Louisiana, for example, shows that bleeding and cupping were not used at all after the 1849–54 cholera epidemic. In 1866, the doses of the still inevitable calomel had decreased. Leland A. Langridge, "Asiatic Cholera in Louisiana, 1832–73" (unpublished Master's thesis Louisiana State University, 1955), pp. 124, 128.

tients who did best had merely been kept warm and given no medication aside from a bit of wine or broth. Reinforcing this bitter experience with cholera itself was a newly critical spirit, which only in academic medicine resulted in a doctrinaire rejection of traditional remedies (so-called therapeutic nihilism), but which helped in general to promote a more sceptical attitude toward the received truths of earlier generations.

It was no longer sufficient to ask simply whether a remedy was effective in treating symptoms. What, more critical physicians already asked, caused these symptoms, and what, if any, was the effect of a drug on such an underlying cause? The most important problem, they argued, lay in the physiological mechanisms by which a proposed remedy might work. Generations of physicians, for instance, had accepted unquestioningly the idea—derived from the Galenic humoral theory—that calomel acted on the liver. But did it? And if so, how?

Such theoretical niceties were suited to the Harvard and Pennsylvania faculties, to physicians trained in the clinics of Paris, London, or Dublin. They were a long time in trickling down to the ordinary practitioner; he continued to purge, puke, and sweat his patients—though, to be sure, a bit less vigorously than had been his custom.

The increasing mildness of his remedies was, however, due more to the mundane factor of competition than to abstract considerations of scientific method. Regular physicians had to offer a therapy as attractive as that proffered by the homeopaths, hydropaths, eclectics, and botanics with whom they competed. If remedies did not heal, they might at least be pleasant. And it was increasingly difficult to believe that medicines actually did heal. Physicians could not guarantee results; and without such pragmatic justification, Americans could see little reason to grant the regular profession's apparently self-serving demand for a "monopoly" of medical practice. During cholera times, sectarian opponents charged, such demands were not merely selfish, but criminal.

Only after great pressure had been placed on the Metropolitan Board of Health did it grudgingly allow homeopathic physicians even a small role in combating the epidemic.[22] Never had the "small trickery and professional charlatanism" of the regular medical profession been more evident; not only was such behavior unjustified, dissidents claimed, it was contrary to the beliefs of every American. In New York, the Homeopathic Medical Society charged, devotees of their system paid half of the city's taxes and constituted at least 50 per cent of its educated population. Yet this numerous and respectable group was being deprived of its equal rights in the choice of physicians hired by the city.[23] What could be more undemocratic?

The narrow and intolerant views of the regular medical profession were, moreover, a hindrance to the progress of human knowledge. As in 1849, the household idols of American rhetoric were employed in attacking the pretensions of the regulars—and especially the "pitiful sectarian spite and miserable meanness of the American Medical Association."[24] Our banner, declared the president of the Homeopathic Medical Society of Pennsylvania, "is the banner of *progress* and *medical freedom*—theirs . . . are *no progress* and *medical slavery*." Hahnemann suffered the same neglect in 1866 that Harvey and Jenner had in earlier centuries; the medical profession was still a bastion of conservatism. It was not a branch of science— homeopathic physicians appealed knowingly to American

[22] The lay administrators of the Metropolitan Board were initially quite friendly to homeopathy, but were subjected to the pressure of the New York Academy of Medicine, which threatened to withdraw its support from the board should it allow homeopathic physicians to practice in the city's cholera hospitals. Eventually, however, the board did permit these medical dissidents to direct wards at the Battery Barracks and Five Points cholera hospitals.

[23] *New York Eclectic Medical Review,* I (1866), 130. For comments on the undemocratic nature of "medically disfranchising" patrons of homeopathy, cf. *ibid.,* pp. 86–87, 191–92; *Evening Post* (New York), March 1, 1866; Homeopathic Medical Society of New York, *Homeopathy and the Metropolitan Board of Health* (New York, 1866), pp. 3–4; *Hahnemannian Monthly,* II (1866), 405–6.

[24] *Herald of Health,* VI (1865), 59.

values—but rather a "caste institution" having no place among the free institutions of the United States.[25]

As in 1849, it was the better educated and more respectable members of society who provided much of the support for medical sectarianism, a situation no more congenial to the *amour-propre* of the medical profession in 1866 than it had been seventeen years earlier. Horace Greeley, for example, found "medical reform" one of the more socially acceptable of his causes. The establishment, he asserted, of an eclectic medical college

... is a palpable expression of a desire for free thought. Resistance to orthodoxy, I think, is doing good in the world. . . . The men who were stoned to death in their day, and the stones used afterwards to build their monuments, were the men who initiated radical changes, instituted great good.[26]

What American could oppose progress and the scientific advances that made it possible?

The situation of the medical profession was a bleak one. Yet the first signs of the scientific revolution soon to transform it were already discernible in 1866.[27] At the same time, Americans accepted a system of values that would automatically translate the achievements of science into the coin of public esteem. Coming events had already begun to cast their shadows.

[25] James B. Wood, "Annual Address . . . ," *Transactions of the Homeopathic Medical Society of Pennsylvania*, 1867, pp. 27–29; O. Davis, "A Brief Historic Review of Medical Eclecticism," *Transactions of the Eclectic Medical Society of New York*, I (1866), 133–35.

[26] *New York Eclectic Medical Review*, II (1867), 178.

[27] It is worth noting, for example, that in 1866, an American physician for the first time attempted through controlled animal experimentation to discover something of the physiological action of cholera. Robert Bartholow, *Cincinnati Lancet and Observer*, N.S. IX (1866), 658–59.

XIII. CONCLUSION: THE WAY WE LIVE NOW

> Feller citizens—the *tail* of civilization is now exactly where the *front* ears was no mor'n sixty years ago.
>
> A WISCONSIN ORATOR, 1849[1]

It was not until the nineteenth century that cholera invaded the Western Hemisphere. Yet at its first appearance, it represented as much a mystery as had the plague five centuries earlier, for the theoretical resources of the average physician in 1832 were not greatly different from those of his medieval predecessor. By 1866, however, only thirty-four years after their first experience with cholera, even provincial American practitioners were familiar with the names of Snow and Pettenkofer, Liebig and Berzelius.

American medical thought had passed seemingly through centuries rather than decades; new ideas, new assumptions, and new habits of thought had supplanted those dominant forty years before. American physicians readily accepted the discovery of the cholera vibrio in 1883. Many had expected it, for they had been brought step by step to an intellectual position that could readily assimilate it. When, in 1873, cholera attacked the United States for the last time, few physicians clung

[1] Quoted in the *People's Friend* (Covington, Ind.), September 8, 1849.

unreservedly to traditional concepts of disease. The inadequacy of such ideas had become more apparent with each succeeding cholera epidemic. Dozens of communities, large and
small, now utilized the preventive measures which had seemed
to protect New York City in 1866.[2]

Cholera could not have been conquered in 1832. The concepts that enabled Snow to construct a meaningful theory of
its causation, the statistics that helped him in validating his
ideas, the public health organization that could put this knowledge to use, did not exist in 1832.[3] Yet the conditions that nurtured cholera already existed. An urban and industrial material
culture had come into being in a society whose habits of
thought and patterns of collective action had been those of a
simpler, largely rural world.

The achievement of the Metropolitan Board of Health in
the summer of 1866 has a historical significance transcending
its undeniable importance in the development of public medicine. It was one of the first successful responses to a specific
challenge of this new industrial society. So well-conceived a
response could only have been made with ideas and artifacts of
this new society and, equally important, only after its existence
had been accepted. Americans had come to realize that their
nation was like other nations—better than most perhaps, yet no
longer different in kind. The problems of the Old World had
become those of the new. With this realization, the first step
had been taken in finding a solution to these problems.

America had changed in the thirty-four years between 1832
and 1866; new states were created out of wilderness, villages

---

[2] For numerous examples of the application of these methods, see U.S.
President, *The Cholera Epidemic of 1873 in the United States,* Exec. Doc.
No. 95, Part A, 43d Cong., 2d sess.

[3] Without having at his disposal the idea of ferments, of catalysis, and of
disease specificity, it is highly doubtful whether Snow would have been able
to formulate so prescient a theory. Had he by some chance deduced it in
1832, it would have found few believers. Even in 1849, only a few physicians
were ready to accept, or understand completely, his ideas.

grew into cities, cities into metropolises. Railroad and telegraph lines contracted the nation's newly acquired continental dimensions, initiating a uniquely American attitude toward space and time. The labor of Irishmen, Germans, even Chinese had helped to bring about so rapid a transformation. The face of the nation had been altered; the character of its population had shifted as well. These material developments had, inevitably, their counterparts in intellectual changes equally far-reaching.[4] Americans in 1866 looked at a new world—and through new eyes.

Cholera in 1866 was a social problem; in 1832, it had still been, to many Americans, a primarily moral dilemma. Disease had become a consequence of man's interaction with his environment; it was no longer an incident in a drama of moral choice and spiritual salvation. This was not an abrupt change; neither was it a consistent and conscious one. Respectable Americans had not wavered in their theoretical adherence to the ultimate significance of spiritual rather than material goals. We find, between 1832 and 1866, shifts in emphasis, not positive avowals or recantations. That part of men's lives and emotions occupied by matters of the spirit had simply decreased.[5] The circumstances of everyday life were too demanding—and in America's great cities, appalling.

The conditions of tenement life were intolerable. To a generation raised in an atmosphere of militant Protestantism, such evils could not be allowed to exist unchanged. It is no accident

[4] Counterparts, advisedly, not causes or consequences. I have taken the perhaps ingenuous course of ignoring the causal and, to a large extent, the temporal relationships between these material and intellectual changes. This ancient philosophical problem, with its rigidly dichotomous statement, seemed to me one best avoided. The historical, rather than the philosophical, sensibility must conceive of this relationship not as one of cause and effect, but in terms of a "dynamic equilibrium" between intellectual and material change (the categorical distinction between which is, in any case, artificial and ahistorical).

[5] This process was, of course, not limited to the years between 1832 and 1866. One might, with some justice, argue that the intensity of religious feeling in the United States has declined since the first half of the seventeenth century, reaching its present nadir only in our own time.

that many of the leaders in the early public health movement in England as well as in the United States were men of deep religious feeling. Not even so doctrinaire a Benthamite as Edwin Chadwick could escape the all-pervading influence of such moral enthusiasm; it was the spirit of the age.[6] The matter-of-fact meliorism of the Metropolitan Board of Health is not necessarily a symptom of the dissipation of spiritual energies, but rather of these energies having been diverted into new channels.

The means of reform had changed, not necessarily its ends—or so pious Americans could believe. The salvation of man's eternal soul was the only real goal of the church. By 1866, however, it was becoming increasingly apparent that the soul could not be made healthy while the body which housed it was diseased. Chloride of lime, not fasting, brought deliverance from cholera; the cure for pauperism lay in education and housing, not prayers and exhortation. Even clergymen were beginning to think habitually in terms of pragmatic goals and environmental causation. It would not be easy to recapture the piety of an earlier generation; preoccupation with material means meant, inevitably, the decreasing reality of spiritual ends.

Moralism is an essential part of the cultural debris left behind by receding waves of piety. Cholera was, in 1866, still made to serve morality's didactic purposes. The concept of predisposing causes remained part of the theoretical armamentarium of almost every physician, despite the increasingly empirical nature of etiological thought and the correspondingly complete acceptance of the idea of disease specificity. Drink and immorality, as well as foul water and dirty bodies, might be re-

---

[6] As one clerical editorialist put it, the Christian had "not only his own salvation to secure, but he is to be an instrument of the salvation of others. To this end he is bound to enlist in every cause calculated to ameliorate the condition of man, and ultimately to contribute to his eternal peace. . . ." J. M. Bailey, *Morning Star* (Dover, N.H.), XXIV (July 11, 1849), 50. It is apparent that the improving zeal of the Benthamites—even of freethinkers both in England and the United States—was religious in a more than metaphorical sense.

sponsible for contracting cholera. Poverty might not be all one's own doing, but it was nevertheless a condition somehow suspect; the poor were still outside society.

Traditional values were not so easily discarded; conventional morality condemned explicitly the grosser manifestations of American materialism. As temporal considerations assumed an ever larger role even in clerical preoccupations, ministers attacked with increasing intensity the vulgar and antisocial behavior exhibited everywhere about them.[7] Only a few fast-day sermons in 1832 dwelt on the nation's pervading materialism; by 1849, it had become an almost obsessive theme. In 1866, jeremiads directed against the moral enormities of post bellum America had become everyday editorial fare. At the same time, and often in a neighboring column, readers were presented with articles on cholera, paragraph upon paragraph detailing the proper manner of disinfecting privies, but not a word on sin and retribution.

It was in America's great cities that the realities of this new society were most apparent. They could not well be ignored. The Irish, for example, worked in one's kitchen, brushed past one in the crowded streets. They, like the Jews, were identified with city life and hence served as a visible—and almost physically irritating—symbol of change. As the piety and confidence

[7] It is possible, though by no means necessary, to assume that the peculiar intensity of such attacks was a result of the guilt and ambivalence produced by the speaker's own participation in the process of change he deplored. See the interpretation of Jacksonian rhetoric by Marvin Meyers, in *The Jacksonian Persuasion* (Stanford, 1957), or the emphasis placed upon the Protestant heritage of guilt by Stanley Elkins in his interpretation of abolitionism, *Slavery: A Problem in American Institutional and Intellectual Life* (Chicago, 1959). Though perhaps indispensable to the writing of social and intellectual history, I find the conception of a "collective consciousness" upon which such interpretations must be based somehow unsatisfying (particularly in so far as the collective consciousness is motivated by the promptings of an unconscious that conforms neatly to the patterns assigned the individual personality by modern dynamic psychology). In any case, and on a purely objective level, the obvious antipathy of Gilded Age morality to traditional Christian values was sufficient cause for such attacks—especially by a ministry that felt more and more its displacement from the central position that it had, or imagined it had, held in the past.

of an earlier day declined, the presence of such alien groups seemed all the more alarming.[8]

How long could the United States be spared the class strife of urban life in the Old World? The Astor Place riots in 1849, the Draft Riots of 1863, might be a mere foretaste of things to come. Only Christianity, traditionalists asserted, could bridge the gap between opposing classes; by 1866, even this seemed inadequate. The rich and poor living together in great cities found in their physical proximity a constant reminder of the social and economic distances which separated them. The wealthy, unable to find an assured social identity in the institutional stabilities of an earlier day, felt threatened from below. The poor, on the other hand, found in their contacts with the wealthy a recurrent exacerbation of natural discontents.

But cities could not be razed; civilization could not be effaced. The creation of the Metropolitan Board of Health was a recognition of this fact. (Primitivism has won a few theoretical points in its enduring conflict with progress, but has, at least in the United States, been defeated in every practical engagement.)[9] The writers of the statute creating the Metropolitan Board of Health felt no doctrinaire distaste for the material culture of nineteenth-century America. They sought rather to use the resources of that society to end what they felt to be its needless waste of human life. The culture that produced New York's slums, produced as well the disinfectants, the telegraph, the scientific insights, employed by the Metropolitan Board in its fight against cholera.

Increasing complexity in social and economic organization

[8] The Jews, for example, as an older millenial world view declined and as the evils of materialism seemed to increase, became increasingly the object of American dislike.

[9] To Thomas Jefferson or Benjamin Rush, city life threatened equally men's health and virtue. George Rosen ("Political Order and Human Health in Jeffersonian Thought," *Bulletin of the History of Medicine*, XXVI [1952], 32–44) has clearly delineated the contrast between this Jeffersonian view and the conviction that later replaced it, namely, the assumption that cities and factories could not be done away with and that man's duty was to work within these conditions in order to ameliorate their worst features.

demanded a corresponding expansion in the tasks of public administration. The casual arrangements with which New York had opposed cholera in 1832 and 1849 were no longer adequate in 1866. New knowledge and new convictions had made necessary the creation of a public health board with both greatly increased responsibilities and the authority to fulfil them. Yet the matter-of-fact authoritarianism of this new health board's operations was still, in 1866, the exception rather than the rule in urban administration. Unlike other organs of municipal government, the board was able to provide an absolute justification for its dictates in their identification with the prestige and authority of science.[10]

Scientific values and habits of thought had assumed a new prominence in the American mind.[11] By 1866, the ordered rationalism still characteristic of consciously formal thought in 1832 had been largely replaced by an unashamed empiricism, not only in medical writings, but in sermons and editorials as well. Stylized arguments and formalistic habits of rhetoric were more suited to a stable graded society, for they provided at once symbol and justification of social stratification.

Such distinctions seemed to have no place in the United States in 1866. Membership in a profession, education, not even the perquisites of birth, guaranteed a secure social status. For a number of reasons, the material success that had replaced these older values as a source of social standing could not, in this new society, provide the inner security they had.[12] In the first place, the acceptance of material success as life's ultimate goal offended deeply held ideological commitments: few Americans could escape the conviction that man's highest concerns were spiritual rather than material. (The United States

10 Such arguments, as has already been noted, did not appeal to the lower classes, who took the divine right of science with a grain of salt.

11 I am, of course, using the word "scientific" as a shorthand symbol for a spectrum of ill-defined—though related—values and habits of thought.

12 In this interpretation, I am indebted to the suggestions of David Donald. See, for example, his Harmsworth Lecture, *An Excess of Democracy: The American Civil War and the Social Process* (Oxford, 1960).

was, of course, committed to an ideology that rejected explicit class distinctions.) Second, the acceptance of material standards of success in an open society meant that the wealthy possessed in their riches no guarantee of status: their success could, and was, being duplicated by others. With each assertion of their own position, prosperous Americans became increasingly uneasy, their affirmations more and more blatant. Here, it would seem, were conditions that might nurture class warfare, even revolution; the fear of such strife was very real in American minds in the generation after Appomattox.

Yet the fabric of American society remained—essentially—intact; America's political institutions had, by 1914, become far more responsive to the conditions of a new industrial society. This is the great accomplishment of the generation that governed America in the first dozen years of this century. The discovery of political techniques appropriate to the ordering of this new society, and the assimilation of these techniques into the pattern of existing governmental institutions, was a task far more complex than the comparatively simple one of preventing cholera.

Progressivism was, if anything, a strategy for the achievement of ordered social change. Many Americans had become convinced that some adjustments would have to be made in the forms of the nation's political life; few, however, wished to alter the essential structure of American society. The problem then was to find the means through which these necessary yet limited changes might be effected. A solution was quickly found: the values and techniques, the habits of mind, produced by a scientific, industrial society constituted a natural implement with which to formulate and to accomplish such social change. Expertise, efficiency, disinterested inquiry were the means by which social injustice might be approached—not as an indictment of American society as a whole, but as a series of specific solvable problems. Few men in the age of Theodore Roosevelt doubted that science could provide the men and the methods with which society might be understood—and con-

ANNOTATED BIBLIOGRAPHY

There is no bibliographical guide to American social history; nor is there such a guide to the history of American medicine. These few pages cannot claim to fill these needs. I hope, however, to have provided the curious reader with some idea of the materials used in the writing of this book and to have, perhaps, saved some unnecessary labor for those who may follow in the same vineyards.

GENERAL BIBLIOGRAPHICAL AIDS

Two American journals—the *Bulletin of the History of Medicine* and the *Journal of the History of Medicine and Allied Sciences*—regularly publish articles on the history of American medicine, though contributions relating to this field are likely to appear in any one of a hundred other journals. Fortunately, the work of the historian has been immeasurably lightened by the efforts of persevering indexers. Since 1939, the *Bulletin of the History of Medicine* has published an annual "Bibliography of the History of Medicine in the United States and Canada." More comprehensive is *Current Work in Medical History*, an indispensable index covering the world's scholarly literature and published quarterly by the Wellcome Historical Medical Library, London. The several series of the *Index-Catalogue of the Library of the Surgeon General's Office* provide an excellent—if unaccountably neglected—source not only for the history of medicine, but for many aspects of American social and intellectual history. Students of the history of religion in America have now available to them the invaluable bibliography compiled by Nelson R. Burr, *A Critical Bibliography of Religion in America*, Vol. IV of *Religion in American Life*, ed. James Ward Smith and A. Leland Jamison (Princeton N.J.: Princeton University Press, 1961).

MANUSCRIPT SOURCES

The most important manuscript source for this study has been the New York City Clerk's Papers, deposited at the Municipal Archives and Records Center, a branch of the New York Public Library. These papers include the minutes books of the Board of Health from June 5, 1829, to November 23, 1836, and from December 8, 1848, to July 2, 1860. File Drawers U-57 to U-60 contain the filed papers of the Board of Health. The approved and filed papers—two separate categories of material—of the Common Council for the years 1832, 1849, and 1866 include reports, resolutions, and petitions relating to the cholera epidemics. The minutes of the Special Medical Committee and the Executive Committee of the Board for 1832, as well as the minutes of the Sanatory Committee of the board for 1849, are also available at the Municipal Archives and Records Center.

The minutes of the Metropolitan Board of Health from March 2, 1866, to September 28, 1868, are in the care of the Secretary of the New York City Department of Health, 125 Worth Street. The papers of the Metropolitan Board have, apparently, not survived. The same, unfortunately, can be said of the papers of Boston, Philadelphia, and Cincinnati. The Boston Medical Library has, however, come into possession of a cholera hospital register dating from 1849, while three similar registers—dating from 1832—may be consulted at the Library of the College of Physicians of Philadelphia. Similar admission ledgers for New York City's cholera hospitals have also proved useful, as they record the age, occupation, and place of birth of those admitted—as well as their temperance or intemperance. These ledgers are also available at the Municipal Archives and Records Center.

The Library of the College of Physicians of Philadelphia contains as well a scrapbook of letters addressed during the summer of 1832 to Professor Samuel Jackson, inquiring as to the nature and treatment of cholera. At the Pennsylvania Historical Society, the diary of Deborah Norris Logan was of particular interest, as were the hastily scrawled diary comments of Dr. William Darrach made during the 1832 epidemic. The Rare Book Room of the New York Academy of Medicine possesses a manuscript account of the cholera epidemic of 1832 by Dr. John Stearn, and a notebook in the hand of Dr. Samuel Smith Purple containing clippings and comments on the 1849 epidemic. The Shattuck, Warren, and Dana papers proved most rewarding of those available at the Massachusetts Historical Society. The Caleb B. Smith papers at the Library of Congress contain many accounts of the epidemic, while the William E. Chandler papers (Vol. 88) contain a revealing sampling of letters on immigration and the danger from cholera in 1892–93. Particularly valuable in formulating a picture of life in nineteenth-century New York City were six volumes of typed transcripts from printed sources "relating to the Social History of New York City," donated to the library by I. N. Phelps Stokes. The Beekman Family papers and the Philip Hone diary deposited at the New York Historical Society also provided illuminating descriptions of the New York epidemics. A number of significant letters relating specifically to New York's brush with cholera in 1832 may be found in the Roosevelt papers at the General Theological Seminary.

PUBLIC DOCUMENTS

Cities and states published numerous special documents relating to cholera and almost always a report on the activities of their board of health during the epidemic. These usually included narrative histories of the epidemic and often the reports of hospital physicians and others employed by boards of health. Though scores were printed, I have listed only those of greatest importance.

Boston. *Report of the Committee of Internal Health on the Asiatic Cholera, Together with a Report of the City Physician on the Cholera Hospital.* Boston: J. H. Eastburn, 1849.

Chicago. *Report of the Board of Health of the City of Chicago, for 1867, 1868, and 1869; and a Sanitary History of Chicago, from 1833 to 1870.* Chicago: Lakeside Publishing Co., 1871.

New York City. *Report of the Proceedings of the Sanatory Committee of the Board of Health, in Relation to the Cholera*

as It Prevailed in New York in 1849. New York: McSpedon &
Baker, 1849.

——. *Reports of Hospital Physicians and Other Documents in
Relation to the Epidemic Cholera of 1832,* ed. DUDLEY ATKINS.
New York: G., C., and M. Carvill, 1832.

NEW YORK STATE. *Annual Report of the Metropolitan Board of
Health, 1866.* New York: C. S. Wescott, 1867.

PHILADELPHIA. *Statistics of Cholera: With the Sanitary Measures
Adopted by the Board of Health, prior to and during the Preva-
lence of the Epidemic in Philadelphia, in the Summer of 1849.*
Philadelphia: King & Baird, 1849.

ROCHESTER, NEW YORK. *Report of the Board of Health, on
Cholera, as It Appeared in Rochester, New York, in 1852.*
Rochester: The Board, 1852.

U. S. HOUSE OF REPRESENTATIVES. *Cholera Morbus.* Report No.
226. 22d Cong., 1st sess., January 20, 1832.

U. S. PRESIDENT. *The Cholera Epidemic of 1873 in the United
States.* Exec. Doc. No. 95, 43d Cong., 2d sess. Washington:
Government Printing Office, 1875.

NEWSPAPERS

Nineteenth-century American newspapers, even those in large
·cities, had often a personal and immediate quality refreshingly
unfamiliar to one accustomed to the characterless fare provided by
mid-twentieth-century journalism. Not only did editors and cor-
respondents comment in passing on the social assumptions and
intellectual preoccupations of their day; newspaper columns were
the vehicles for essays, poems, sermons, for the disquisitions generally, of the educated and articulate. Medical articles, for example, of an impressively technical sort were often printed in newspapers. Though historians are frequent users of newspaper sources,
they tend to cite again and again the same newspapers—those
which, like the New York *Times* or Albany *Argus*, have already
become part of our tradition of historical scholarship. Religious
newspapers are infrequently consulted as are small town and provincial papers, while most social and intellectual historians make
comparatively little use of newspaper sources.

The most influential religious newspapers of this period, at least judged by the frequency with which they were quoted and referred to, were *Zion's Herald* and the *Christian Watchman-Examiner* in Boston, and in New York the *Evangelist* and *Christian Advocate*. After its founding in the winter of 1848–49, the *Independent* soon became the most widely read of such papers. The older general and historical libraries have often surprisingly good collections of religious papers. Many such papers, however, are available only in specialized libraries. An excellent collection of Presbyterian newspapers, for example, may be consulted at the Presbyterian Historical Society in Philadelphia, while an equally extensive collection of Episcopalian papers has been preserved at New York's General Theological Seminary. Union Theological Seminary also has a representative collection of such publications.

Particularly difficult of access are the opinions of the less educated and less articulate. Much can be extrapolated from the editorial stance of those metropolitan newspapers that consciously appealed to "popular" sentiments. The social opinions of the Catholic press are often valuable in this connection. Unfortunately, Catholic newspapers were not numerous in this period. (The best collection of such publications is available at Catholic University of America in Washington.)

Special-interest newspapers, often weeklies, are usually classed by librarians as serials, though their nineteenth-century format was that of newspapers. They are, accordingly, not listed in the *Union List of Newspapers* and are thus difficult to locate unless one knows their precise titles. The following list includes all such publications used in this study. General newspapers are much easier to locate, and I have not chosen to list those which I consulted; the text notes provide an adequate reflection of their titles and places of publication.

Connecticut, Hartford
  Christian Secretary. 1866. (Baptist.)
  Connecticut Churchman. 1866. (Episcopal.)
  Connecticut Observer. 1832. (Congregational.)
  Episcopal Watchman. 1832.
District of Columbia
  National Era. 1849. (Antislavery.)

Illinois, Chicago
  Christian Times and Witness. 1866. (Baptist.)
  Herald of the Prairies. 1849. (Interdenominational: "Evangelical.")
  North-Western Presbyterian. 1866.
Kentucky, Lexington
  Western Luminary. 1832–33. (Presbyterian.)
Kentucky, Louisville
  Baptist Banner. 1849.
  Examiner. 1849. (Antislavery.)
  Free Christian Commonwealth. 1866. (Presbyterian.)
  Presbyterian Herald. 1849.
Maine, Gardiner
  Christian Intelligencer and Eastern Chronicle. 1832. (Universalist.)
Maine, Limerick
  Morning Star. 1832. (Freewill Baptist.)
Maine, Portland
  Christian Mirror. 1832, 1849, 1866. (Congregationalist.)
Maryland, Baltimore
  Catholic Mirror. 1866.
  Katholische Volksveitung. 1865–66.
Massachusetts, Boston
  Boston Investigator. August 23, 1848–49, 1866. (Freethought.)
  Boston Pilot. 1849, 1866. (Catholic.)
  Boston Recorder. 1832, 1849. (Congregational.) Title changes to *Puritan Recorder*, June 7, 1849.
  Christian Register. 1832, 1849, 1866. (Unitarian.)
  Christian Watchman & Reflector. 1866. (Baptist.) See *Watchman-Examiner*.
  Christian Witness and Church Advocate. 1849. (Episcopal.)
  Congregationalist. June–December, 1849.
  Liberator. 1849. (Antislavery.)
  Olive Branch. 1849. (Congregationalist.)
  Trumpet and Universalist Magazine. 1832, 1849, 1866. Title varies.
  Watchman-Examiner. 1832, 1849, 1866. (Baptist.) Title varies.
  Zion's Herald and Wesleyan Journal. 1849, 1866. (Methodist.)

Massachusetts, Milford
  Practical Christian. 1849.
Massachusetts, Worcester
  Burritt's Christian Citizen. December 2, 1848–September, 1849.
New Hampshire, Dover
  Morning Star. 1849. (Freewill Baptist.)
New York, Hempstead
  Inquirer. 1832. (Freethought.)
New York, New York
  Age of Reason. 1849. (Freethought.)
  America's Own. April, 1849–December, 1849. (Radical, anti-
    clerical.)
  Christian Advocate. 1832, 1849, 1866. (Methodist.)
  Christian Ambassador. 1848–49. (Universalist.)
  Christian Intelligencer. 1832, 1849, 1866. (Dutch Reformed.)
  Christian Messenger. 1832. (Universalist.)
  Churchman. 1832, 1849. (Episcopal.)
  Evangelist. 1832, 1849, 1866. (Presbyterian.)
  Free Enquirer. 1832. (Freethought.)
  Freeman's Journal and Catholic Register. 1849, 1866.
  Independent. 1849, 1866. (Congregational.)
  Independent Beacon. 1849–50. (Freethought, associationist.)
  Irish American. 1866.
  Jewish Messenger. 1866.
  Methodist. 1866.
  New-York Recorder. 1849. (Baptist.)
  New-York Observer. 1832, 1849, 1866. (Presbyterian.)
  Presbyterian. 1849, 1866.
  Protestant Churchman. 1849. (Episcopal.)
  Sentinel. 1832. (Radical, freethought.) See the *Workingman's
    Advocate* for weekly edition.
  Truth Teller. 1832. (Catholic.)
  Workingman's Advocate. 1832.
New York, Rochester
  Liberal Advocate. 1832–33 (Freethought.)
New York, Utica
  Evangelical Magazine and Gospel Advocate. 1832. (Universalist.)
Ohio, Cincinnati
  Baptist Weekly Journal of the Mississippi Valley. 1832.
  Catholic Telegraph. 1832, 1849, 1866.

Central Watchman. 1849. (Presbyterian.)

Cincinnati Journal. 1832. (Presbyterian.) Title varies; see also *Western Luminary.*

Israelite. 1866. Title changes to *American Israelite.*

Presbyter. 1866.

Standard. 1832. (Presbyterian.)

Wahrheitsfreund. 1849. 1866. (Catholic.)

Western Christian Advocate. 1849. (Methodist.)

Ohio, Hudson

Ohio Observer. 1849. (Congregationalist.)

Pennsylvania, Chambersburg

German Reformed Weekly Messenger. 1849, 1866.

Pennsylvania, Philadelphia

American Presbyterian and Genesee Evangelist. 1866.

Catholic Herald. 1849.

Christian Observer. 1849. (Presbyterian.)

Philadelphia Liberalist. 1832. (Universalist.)

Philadelphian. 1832. (Presbyterian.)

Pennsylvania, Pittsburgh

Christian Herald. 1832. (Presbyterian.)

Pittsburgh Catholic. 1849, 1866.

Presbyterian Banner. 1866.

South Carolina, Charleston

Charleston Observer. 1832. (Presbyterian.)

Southern Christian Advocate. 1849. (Methodist.)

Tennessee, Nashville

Presbyterian Record. 1849.

Vermont, Windsor

Vermont Chronicle. 1832. (Presbyterian.)

Vermont, Woodstock

Universalist Watchman, Repository and Chronicle. 1832.

Virginia, Richmond

Christian Observer. 1866. (Presbyterian.)

Religious Herald. 1849, 1866. (Baptist.)

Watchman and Observer. 1866. (Presbyterian.)

Wisconsin, Milwaukee

Wisconsin Free Democrat. 1849. (Antislavery.)

Volksfreund. 1849. (Freethought.)

PRINTED SOURCES: MEDICAL

Between 1873 and 1875, John Shaw Billings directed the preparation of a bibliography on cholera. When completed, it ran to
some three hundred pages and in its accuracy and inclusiveness
marked a minor landmark in the history of medical bibliography.
(It was published as Part C, pp. 708–1025, of *The Cholera Epidemic of 1873 in the United States*, Exec. Doc. No. 95 [Washing-
ton, 1875].)

I have, with a few exceptions, read everything in this bibliography pertaining to cholera in the United States between 1832 and
1866, as well as some of the more important and influential European publications. Most of these articles were of no particular
merit; and in view of the availability of the Billings bibliography,
it would be a needless task to attempt to list them in any formal
fashion. The more important or interesting items are mentioned
in the text and notes—and discussed in some greater detail in my
article, "The Cause of Cholera: Aspects of Etiological Thought
in Nineteenth Century America," *Bulletin of the History of Medicine*, XXXIV (July–August, 1960), 331–54. Many of the classic
papers in the development of our knowledge of the disease have
been conveniently listed and excerpted by Arthur Bloomfield, in
A Bibliography of Internal Medicine: Communicable Diseases.
(Chicago: University of Chicago Press, 1958), pp. 17–32.

In the period between 1832 and 1866, the most important American medical journal was the *American Journal of the Medical
Sciences* (Philadelphia). This appeared quarterly and printed the
lengthier and more ambitious articles of American physicians.
Widely read, especially in New England, was the *Boston Medical
and Surgical Journal*, a weekly with more editorial and news
matter. These were only two, however, among dozens of such
journals. There are excellent collections of such nineteenth-century medical serials in the National Library of Medicine and the
New York Academy of Medicine. These are easily the two out-
standing collections in the country, though both the Boston Medical Library and the Library of the College of Physicians of Philadelphia are adequate. During the 1832 epidemic, physicians in
New York and Philadelphia published, respectively, the *Cholera
Bulletin* and the *Cholera Gazette*. Though ephemeral, both contained much valuable material. Transactions of state and local

medical societies are also a most useful source, often including addresses, reports and other programmatic statements—as well as the comments they provoked from the floor.

The sectarian journals, those published by hydropaths, eclectics, homeopaths, and the like, are often difficult to locate. Such publications were ignored by "regular" medical libraries; and the schools that taught these dissident beliefs have been closed and their libraries dispersed. The National Library of Medicine has, fortunately, a representative collection of such journals; and the library of the New York Medical College possesses an excellent collection of homeopathic publications. Most of my references to the writings of homeopaths come from the holdings of these libraries. A bibliography and union list of such unconventional medical publications would be a most valuable aid to the medical and social historian.

PRINTED MATERIALS OTHER THAN MEDICAL

It would be pointless to list all those printed diaries, journals, memoirs, and collections of letters in which references to cholera were found. A few, however, were of particular relevance, and I have listed them below. Most of my conclusions regarding the religious interpretations of the epidemic were garnered from the religious newspapers, which were usually edited by ministers and whose pages often provided the final resting place for lectures and sermons. Some sermons, however, were printed separately, and the list following includes the more interesting and representative of these.

ALGER, WILLIAM R. *Inferences from the Pestilence and the Fast: A Discourse Preached in the Mount Pleasant Congregational Church, Roxbury, Mass., August 3, 1849.* Boston: Crosby & Nichols, 1849.

ALLEN, J. H. *A Sermon on the Coming of the Cholera, Preached in the Unitarian Church, Washington, June 10, 1849.* Washington, D.C.: J. and G. S. Gideon, 1849.

ALLEN, LEWIS F. "First Appearance, in 1832, of the Cholera in Buffalo," *Transactions of the Buffalo Historical Society*, IV (1896), 245–56.

AMERICAN TRACT SOCIETY. *An Appeal on the Subject of Cholera to the Prepared and Unprepared.* New York: The Society, 1832.

ARNOLD, RICHARD D. *Letters of Richard D. Arnold, M.D., 1808–1876*, ed. RICHARD H. SHRYOCK. ("Papers of the Trinity College Historical Society," Double Series XVIII–XIX.) Durham, N.C.: Trinity College Historical Society, 1929.

BARNES, ALBERT. "The Pestilence," *American National Preacher.* XXIII (September, 1849), 197–213.

BARRETT, SAMUEL. *A Sermon Preached in the Twelfth Congregational Church, Boston, Thursday, August 9, 1832. The Day Appointed for Fasting, Humiliation, and Prayer, on Account of the Approach of the Cholera.* Boston: Hilliard, Gray & Co., 1832.

BEMAN, NATHAN. *The Influence of Ardent Spirits in the Production of Cholera.* Troy, N.Y.: Troy Sentinel Office, 1832.

BOWDITCH, VINCENT Y. *Life and Correspondence of Henry Ingersoll Bowditch.* 2 vols. Boston: Houghton Mifflin, 1902.

CARUTHERS, WILLIAM A. *The Kentuckian in New-York. Or, the Adventures of Three Southerns.* 2 vols. New York: Harper & Brothers, 1834.

CHALMERS, THOMAS. *The Efficacy of Prayer. A Sermon Preached at St. George's Church, Edinburgh, on Thursday, March 22, 1832. . . .* 2d ed. Boston: Clapp & Hull, 1832.

CHEEVER, HENRY T. "God's Meaning in Men's Suffering," *American National Preacher*, XXIII (June, 1849), 125–37.

CLAPP, THEODORE. *Autobiographical Sketches and Recollections, during a Thirty-five Years' Residence in New Orleans.* 3d ed. Boston: Phillips, Sampson & Co., 1858.

DEWEY, ORVILLE. *A Sermon on the Moral Uses of the Pestilence, Denominated Asiatic Cholera. Delivered on Fast-Day, August 9, 1832.* New Bedford, Mass.: Benj. T. Congdon, 1832.

DIXON, EDWARD H. *Scenes in the Practice of a New York Surgeon.* New York: DeWitt & Davenport, 1855.

DUNLAP, WILLIAM. *Diary of William Dunlap (1766–1839).* ("Collections of the New York Historical Society for the Year 1931.") 3 vols. New York: The Society, 1930.

FINNEY, CHARLES GRANDISON. *Memoirs of Rev. Charles G. Finney.* New York: A. S. Barnes & Co., 1876.

FREEMAN, J. M. "New York City as a Mission Field," *Methodist*, VI (December 23, 1865), 401; VI (December 30, 1865), 409.

GREENWOOD, F. W. F. *Prayer for the Sick. A Sermon Preached at King's Chapel, Boston, on Thursday, August 9, 1832.* . . . Boston: Leonard C. Bowles, 1832.

HONE, PHILIP. *The Diary of Philip Hone, 1828–1851.* 2 vols. New York: Dodd, Mead & Co., 1927.

JACKSON, JAMES. *A Memoir of James Jackson, Jr., M.D., with Extracts from His Letters to His Father; and Medical Cases, Collected by Him.* Boston: I. R. Butts, 1835.

LESSER, ISAAC. "The Plague," *Occident,* VII (September, 1849), 289–301.

NOBLE, MASON. *A Sermon Delivered in the Fourth Presbyterian Church in the City of Washington, on a Day of Thanksgiving (November 22, 1832) for the Departure of the Cholera from That City.* Washington, D.C.: J. Gideon, 1832.

PALFREY, JOHN G. *A Discourse Delivered in the Church in Brattle Square, Boston, August 9, 1832.* . . . Boston: Gray and Bowen, 1832.

PINTARD, JOHN. *Letters from John Pintard to His Daughter Eliza Noel Pintard Davidson, 1816–1833.* ("Collections of the New York Historical Society for the Year 1940.") 4 vols. New York: The Society, 1941.

SPRING, GARDINER. *A Sermon Preached August 3, 1832, a Day Set Apart in the City of New-York for Public Fasting, Humiliation, and Prayer, on Account of the Malignant Cholera.* New York: Jonathan Leavitt, 1832.

STRONG, GEORGE TEMPLETON. *The Diary of George Templeton Strong, 1835–1875,* ed. ALLAN NEVINS and MILTON HALSEY THOMAS. 4 vols. New York: Macmillan, 1952.

THAYER, CHRISTOPHER. *A Discourse Delivered in the First Church, Beverly, at the Fast Observed in Massachusetts on Account of the Prevailing Cholera, August 9, 1832.* Salem, Mass.: Foote and Brown, 1832.

TUFTS, MARSHALL. *A History of the Cholera; the Universal Epidemic and Scourge of Mankind; Its Claims to Distinction as a Providential Dispensation; and a Comparative View of Former Epidemics.* Lexington, Mass., 1833.

WALKER, AUGUSTUS. "Early Days on the Lakes, with an Account of the Cholera Visitation of 1832," *Transactions of the Buffalo Historical Society,* V (1902), 287–318.

WILSON, JOSEPH G. *The Voice of God in the Storm, A Discourse Delivered in the Presbyterian Church, on the Day of the National Fast, August 3, 1849.* Lafayette, Ind.: Rosser & Bros., 1849.

SECONDARY SOURCES

One interested in learning something further of nineteenth-century medicine could begin at no better place than Knud Faber's *Nosography,* an uncommonly lucid essay on the development of modern internal medicine. (Complete citations will be found in the list of sources immediately following this text.) The pertinent chapters in Ackerknecht's *Short History of Medicine* and Shryock's *Development of Modern Medicine* present contrasting overviews of the period. The modern literature on cholera is well summarized in Pollitzer's recent study of *Cholera,* which contains moreover an excellent historical introduction.

There is, unfortunately, no comprehensive recent history of American medicine. The standard older history by Francis Packard is not always reliable as to detail and lacks any organizing principle. The best history of American medicine is that to be found in the articles and books of Richard H. Shryock. The text notes to his lectures on *Medicine and Society in America, 1660–1860* provide a useful, if informal, guide to the bibliography of this period. There is much state and local history of American medicine, varying greatly in quality, but nevertheless a valuable source of information. Undoubtedly the most useful of these is Wyndham Blanton's three-volume history of medicine in Virginia. Few professional historians have devoted their efforts to such local history, though two recent monographs by Thomas Bonner on medicine in Chicago and Kansas are valuable exceptions to this generalization.

Historians have, however, been attracted to particular aspects of American medical history. The articles and unpublished dissertation of Alex Berman present a detailed account of the history of botanic medicine in this country. (Unfortunately, there is no comparable study of either homeopathy or hydropathy, though the materials for such a history are abundant.) H. B. Shafer's thorough study of the *American Medical Profession, 1783 to 1850,* is still valuable and may profitably be read in connection with Donald Konold's "History of American Medical Ethics." A more complete history of the American medical profession is badly needed. William T. Norwood's history of *Medical Education in the United States before the Civil War* is indispensable though narrow in perspective. Leonard K. Eaton's study of *New England Hospitals* illustrates how much can be drawn from the imaginative analysis of a narrowly defined subject. George Rosen's recent survey of the *History of Public Health* provides an excellent place to begin for one interested in the social and economic implications of public medicine. The most vivid accounts of nineteenth-century American medicine are still those written by participants; the autobiographies of Charles Caldwell, Benjamin Rush, and Samuel D. Gross are indispensable sources for the study of this period. An interesting and well-written introduction to the history of theories of disease causation is provided by C.-E. A. Winslow in *Conquest of Epidemic Disease*. William Bulloch's *History of Bacteriology* is detailed and reliable; more recent references can be found in Thomas H. Grainger's *Guide to the History of Bacteriology*. Excellent, but unfortunately brief, is Arthur Hughes's *History of Cytology*.

Deferring to the existence of Nelson Burr's *Critical Bibliography of Religion in America*, let me note briefly only those few books that have been most influential in forming my interpretation of American religion in mid-nineteenth century. These are the *Burned-over District*, by Whitney Cross, and the studies by Perry Miller on *The New England Mind* and Conrad Wright on the *Beginnings of Unitarianism*. There are, as well, invaluable references in Arthur A. Ekirch's study of the *Idea of Progress in America* and Albert Post's monograph on *Popular Freethought in America, 1825–1850*.

ABELL, AARON I. *The Urban Impact on American Protestantism, 1865–1900*. ("Harvard Historical Studies," Vol. LXV.) Cambridge, Mass.: Harvard University, 1943.

ACKERKNECHT, ERWIN H. *Malaria in the Upper Mississippi Valley, 1860–1900*. (Supplements to the *Bulletin of the History of Medicine*, No. 4.) Baltimore: Johns Hopkins University, 1945.

———. "Anticontagionism between 1821 and 1867," *Bulletin of the History of Medicine*, XXII (September–October, 1948), 562–93.

————. "Hygiene in France, 1815–1848," *Bulletin of the History of Medicine*, XXII (April, 1948), 117–55.

————. *A Short History of Medicine*. New York: Ronald Press Co., 1955.

ALBION, ROBERT, with the collaboration of JENNIE BARNES POPE. *The Rise of New York Port (1815–1860)*. New York: Charles Scribner's Sons, 1939.

ALLEN, PHYLLIS. "Americans and the Germ Theory of Disease." Unpublished doctoral thesis, University of Pennsylvania, 1949.

ATKINS, GORDON. *Health, Housing, and Poverty in New York City, 1865–1898*. Garden City, N.Y.: The author, 1947.

BERMAN, ALEX. "The Impact of the Nineteenth-century Botanico-Medical Movement in American Pharmacy and Medicine." Unpublished doctoral thesis, University of Wisconsin, 1954.

————. "The Thomsonian Movement and Its Relation to American Pharmacy and Medicine," *Bulletin of the History of Medicine*, XXV (September–October, 1951), 405–28; *ibid.*, XXV (November–December, 1951), 519–38.

————. "Social Roots of the 19th Century Botanico-Medical Movement in the United States," *Actes du VIIIe Congrès International d'Histoire des Sciences* (Florence, September 3–9, 1956), pp. 561–65.

BILLINGTON, RAY ALLEN. *The Protestant Crusade, 1800–1860: A Study of the Origins of American Nativism*. New York: Macmillan, 1938.

BLAKE, NELSON M. *Water for the Cities: A History of the Urban Water Supply Problem in the United States*. Syracuse, N.Y.: Syracuse University, 1956.

BLANTON, WYNDHAM B. *Medicine in Virginia in the Nineteenth Century*. Richmond: Garrett & Massie, 1933.

BODO, JOHN R. *The Protestant Clergy and Public Issues 1812–1848*. Princeton, N.J.: Princeton University, 1954.

BONNER, THOMAS NEVILLE. *Medicine in Chicago, 1850–1950: A Chapter in the Social and Scientific Development of a City*. Madison, Wis.: American History Research Center, 1957.

BREMNER, ROBERT H. *From the Depths: The Discovery of Poverty in the United States*. New York: New York University, 1956.

BULLOCH, WILLIAM. *The History of Bacteriology*. London: Oxford, 1938.

CHAMBERS, J. S. *The Conquest of Cholera*. New York: Macmillan, 1938.

CHEVALIER, LOUIS. *Le Choléra, La première épidémie du XIXe siècle*. (Bibliothèque de la révolution de 1848. Tome XX.) Le Roche: Impr. Centrale de l'ouest, 1958.

COLE, CHARLES C., JR. *The Social Ideas of the Northern Evangelists, 1826–1860*. New York: Columbia University, 1954.

CROSS, WHITNEY R. *The Burned-over District: The Social and Intellectual History of Enthusiastic Religion in Western New York, 1800–1850*. Ithaca, N.Y.: Cornell University, 1950.

DONALD, DAVID. *An Excess of Democracy: The American Civil War and the Social Process*. Oxford: Oxford University, 1960.

DUFFY, JOHN. *Epidemics in Colonial America*. Baton Rouge: Louisiana State University, 1953.

EATON, LEONARD K. *New England Hospitals, 1790–1833*. Ann Arbor: University of Michigan, 1957.

EKIRCH, ARTHUR A. *The Idea of Progress in America, 1815–1860*. New York: Columbia University, 1944.

ERNST, ROBERT. *Immigrant Life in New York City, 1825–1863*. New York: King's Crown, 1949.

FABER, KNUD. *Nosography: The Evolution of Clinical Medicine in Modern Times*. With an introductory note by RUFUS COLE, M.D. 2d ed. revised. New York: Paul B. Hoeber, 1930.

GRAINGER, THOMAS H. *A Guide to the History of Bacteriology*. New York: Ronald Press, 1958.

GRIFFIN, CLIFFORD S. *Their Brothers' Keepers: Moral Stewardship in the United States, 1800–1865*. New Brunswick, N.J.: Rutgers University, 1960.

HANDLIN, OSCAR. *Boston's Immigrants: A Study in Acculturation*. 2d ed. revised. Boston: Harvard University, 1959.

HIGHAM, JOHN. *Strangers in the Land: Patterns of American Nativism, 1860–1925*. New Brunswick, N.J.: Rutgers University, 1955.

HUGHES, ARTHUR. *A History of Cytology*. London: Abelard-Schuman, 1959.

KONOLD, DONALD E. "A History of American Medical Ethics, 1847–1912." Unpublished doctoral thesis, University of Missouri, 1954.

KRAMER, HOWARD D. "Early Municipal and State Boards of Health," *Bulletin of the History of Medicine*, XXIV (November–December, 1950), 503–29.

———. "The Beginnings of the Public Health Movement in the United States," *Bulletin of the History of Medicine*, XXI (May–June, 1947), 352–76.

LANGRIDGE, LELAND A. "Asiatic Cholera in Louisiana, 1832–73." Unpublished Master's thesis, Louisiana State University, 1955.

LUBOVE, ROY. "The Progressives and the Slums: Tenement House Reform in New York City, 1890–1917." Unpublished doctoral thesis, Cornell University, 1960.

MACLEAR, JAMES FULTON. " 'The True American Union' of Church and State: The Reconstruction of the Theocratic Tradition," *Church History*, XXVIII (March, 1959), 3–24.

McLOUGHLIN, WILLIAM G. "Introduction," in *Lectures on Revivals of Religion*, by CHARLES GRANDISON FINNEY. Cambridge, Mass.: Harvard University, 1960. Pp. vii–lii.

MILLER, PERRY. *The New England Mind*. 2 vols. Cambridge, Mass.: Harvard University, 1939, 1953.

NORWOOD, WILLIAM T. *Medical Education in the United States before the Civil War*. With a foreword by HENRY E. SIGERIST. Philadelphia: University of Pennsylvania, 1944.

PACKARD, FRANCIS R. *History of Medicine in the United States*. 2 vols. New York: Paul E. Hoëber, 1931.

PECKHAM, HOWARD H. "Tears for Old Tippecanoe: Religious Interpretations of President Harrison's Death," *Proceedings of the American Antiquarian Society* (April, 1959), pp. 17–36.

POST, ALBERT. *Popular Freethought in America, 1825–1850*. New York: Columbia University, 1943.

POWELL, J. H. *Bring Out Your Dead*. Philadelphia: University of Pennsylvania, 1949.

ROSEN, GEORGE. "What Is Social Medicine? A Genetic Analysis of the Concept," *Bulletin of the History of Medicine*, XXI (September–October, 1947), 674–733.

———. "Political Order and Human Health in Jeffersonian Thought," *Bulletin of the History of Medicine*, XXVI (January–February, 1952), 32–44.

———. "The Fate of the Concept of Medical Police, 1780–1890," *Centaurus*, V, No. 1 (1957), 97–113.

ROSENBERG, CHARLES. "The Cholera Epidemic of 1832 in New York City," *Bulletin of the History of Medicine*, XXXIII (January–February, 1959), 37–49.

———. "The Cause of Cholera: Aspects of Etiological Thought in Nineteenth Century America," *Bulletin of the History of Medicine*, XXXIV (July–August, 1960), 331–54.

SCHNEIDER, DAVID. *The History of Public Welfare in New York State, 1609–1866*. Chicago: University of Chicago, 1938.

SHRYOCK, RICHARD H. "Public Relations of the Medical Profession in Great Britain and the United States: 1600–1870," *Annals of Medical History*, N.S. II (May, 1930), 308–38.

———. *American Medical Research Past and Present*. New York: Commonwealth Fund, 1947.

———. *The Development of Modern Medicine: An Interpretation of the Social and Scientific Factors Involved*. New York: Alfred A. Knopf, 1947.

———. *Medicine and Society in America, 1660–1860*. New York: New York University, 1960.

SMITH, TIMOTHY L. *Revivalism and Social Reform in Mid-Nineteenth-Century America*. New York: Abingdon Press, 1957.

STEVENSON, LLOYD G. "Science Down the Drain," *Bulletin of the History of Medicine*, XXIX (January–February, 1955), 1–26.

STOKES, I. N. PHELPS. *The Iconography of Manhattan Island, 1498–1909*. 6 Vols. New York: Robert H. Dodd, 1926.

WALKER, WILLIAM B. "The Health Reform Movement in the United States, 1830–1870." Unpublished doctoral dissertation, Johns Hopkins University, 1955.

WARREN, CHARLES. *Odd Byways in American History*. Cambridge, Mass.: Harvard University, 1942.

WINSLOW, CHARLES-EDWARD AMORY. *Conquest of Epidemic Disease*. Princeton, N.J.: Princeton University, 1943.

WRIGHT, CONRAD. *The Beginnings of Unitarianism in America*. Boston: Starr King, 1955.

YOUNG, JAMES HARVEY. *The Toadstool Millionaires: A Social History of Patent Medicines in America before Federal Regulation*. Princeton, N.J.: Princeton University, 1961.

INDEX